T0220447

Treatment Program Evaluation

This invaluable text provides a rigorous guide to the assessment and evaluation of treatment programs through a multi-disciplinary, holistic model of care. It highlights issues of race, social justice, and health equity, and offers real-world guidance to effect community healing and transformation.

Written by a researcher and experienced evaluator, the book begins by outlining the theories and research which frame our understanding of substance misuse, and upon which treatment programs are based. It then examines the principles which should underpin any evaluation, before detailing the practical various steps required to conduct an evaluation, from data collection to outcome measurement. The book shows, too, through detailed and effective evaluation, policy changes can be made and treatment programs improved. Including practical examples of evaluation and assessment throughout, and also assessing the numerous social systems which can support recovery, the book builds to a four-step public health model for establishing sustainable treatment programs.

In an era where substance misuse has reached epidemic proportions in the United States and beyond, this book will be essential reading for anyone involved in public health policy and practice in this important area.

Allyson Kelley is the principal consultant and founder of Allyson Kelley & Associates PLLC (www.allysonkelleypllc.com). Allyson supports research, evaluation, training, and technical assistance efforts for several community health initiatives in the United States. Her research interests include building community capacity to address the cultural, social, and environmental factors that contribute to differences in health outcomes among underserved populations in the United States. Allyson is committed to building the next generation of public health professionals and has mentored more than 300 undergraduate and graduate students. Allyson's goal is to ensure the voices and expertise of underrepresented organizations and minority groups are published and known. She is the author of two books published by Routledge, *Evaluation in Rural Communities* and *Public Health Evaluation and the Social Determinants of Health*. Allyson earned her Master's degree in Public Health Practice from the University of Alaska Anchorage and her Doctorate in Public Health from the University of North Carolina at Greensboro.

Treatment Program Evaluation
Public Health Perspectives on Mental Health and Substance Use Disorders

Allyson Kelley

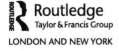
Routledge
Taylor & Francis Group

LONDON AND NEW YORK

Cover image: © Getty Images

First published 2022
by Routledge
4 Park Square, Milton Park, Abingdon, Oxon OX14 4RN

and by Routledge
605 Third Avenue, New York, NY 10158

Routledge is an imprint of the Taylor & Francis Group, an informa business

British Library Cataloguing-in-Publication Data
A catalogue record for this book is available from the British Library

Library of Congress Cataloguing-in-Publication Data
Names: Kelley, Allyson, 1976- author.
Title: Treatment program evaluation : public health perspectives on mental health and substance use disorders / Allyson Kelley.
Description: Milton Park, Abingdon, Oxon ; New York, NY : Routledge, [2022] | Includes bibliographical references and index. |
Identifiers: LCCN 2021059638 (print) | LCCN 2021059639 (ebook) | ISBN 9781032269689 (hardback) | ISBN 9781032148564 (paperback) | ISBN 9781003290728 (ebook) Subjects: LCSH: Public health--Evaluation. | Equality--Health aspects. | Mental illness--Treatment. | Substance abuse--Treatment. |
Classification: LCC RA427 .K297 2022 (print) | LCC RA427 (ebook) | DDC 362.1--dc23/eng/20211221
LC record available at https://lccn.loc.gov/2021059638
LC ebook record available at https://lccn.loc.gov/2021059639

ISBN: 978-1-032-26968-9 (hbk)
ISBN: 978-1-032-14856-4 (pbk)
ISBN: 978-1-003-29072-8 (ebk)

DOI: 10.4324/9781003290728

Typeset in Goudy
by MPS Limited, Dehradun

This book is dedicated to everyone that has lost something because of untreated mental health and substance use disorders... family members, time, friends, money, pride, reputation, trust, and hope. It is time to regain and recover what has been lost. Treatment programs pave the way. They open their doors and welcome all of us in. Evaluators work by their side, wanting, knowing, and seeking evidence about what works, for whom, why, and when. Families and communities provide support every step of the way. This is a recovery generation.

Contents

Figures

Tables

Boxes

Map

Foreword

In the field of substance use/behavioral health a phrase, often used describing the baffling nature of the disease, is to state "Insanity is doing the same thing over and over again, expecting different results." This phrase is used to help convince the individual suffering with the addictive cycle to begin observing their thoughts, and behaviors to make changes.

I think of this phrase when I think about operating programs and offering behavioral health services within a continuum of care without program evaluation and data analysis. Prior to our program's relationship with Allyson Kelley and her evaluation team, we would gather data for reports. This process was very rudimentary and consisted of reporting of numbers. At times, we would use to make programmatic changes, for example no show rates thus making change that connection to folks.

Now, with clearer understanding the benefit of professional program evaluation and data analysis the program is thriving in areas we would not have foreseen. The staff have a distinct understanding of how the direct work they provide has an impact not only with an individual but also programmatically. The process has led to directing program goals, assisting in our vision and recognizing our impact on community within varying aspects of treatment. Staff are being creative and invested. It has quelled the insanity of fitting our community to generalized services. The story being told within our evaluation, survey information and data analysis has shifted the perspective of service delivery. We have gained insight that our approaches to services vary within community needs vary and require inclusiveness. The process lies within the community, and we now trust the process.

Performing this evaluation work within a Public Health model is genius. Operating Behavioral Health/Substance Use services from a strength-based approach, as opposed to a deficit approach, lends to positive Outcomes and drive continued evaluation.

I congratulate Allyson on the decision to write this book which will be used within Academia. However, it should be utilized by programs and agencies within the fields of Human Services to increase services improvements and successes. Evaluation and data analysis is important work. Program Director's should put this as a line item within program budgets for collaborative efforts with professional evaluation.

Much appreciation to Allyson Kelley and her team from our People.

Kellie Webb, LAT,
Program Director, Eastern Shoshone
Recovery Program, Ft Washakie WY

Preface

We all need recovery. One of the most obvious signs of the need for recovery and healing is the high rates of substance abuse and misuse in our world. Untreated addiction and mental health issues are the most glaring, wicked problems of our time. If we ignore these issues, they will not go away, they will continue to claim the lives of mothers, fathers, our children, relatives, friends, and colleagues. But these losses and suffering are not necessary. What is necessary is a fundamental shift in how we approach addiction, treatment, and recovery. We have evidence that individualistic approaches to treatment do not work. A public health approach calls for changing the broader systems and social contexts. What I do know is that treatment programs are leading the way toward a recovery generation. A generation that no longer suffers and believes that healing is possible because they see it every day, in the transformation, hope, and actions of participants and communities involved in recovery.

I organized this book based on my work evaluating treatment programs. Chapter 1 defines the issue of mental health and substance abuse based on United States and global estimates. Drawing from multiple studies and reports, this chapter is a must read for anyone wanting to know more about the problem. Chapter 1 also introduces the concept of a public health approach to the evaluation of treatment programs. The first step in a public health approach is defining the problem, hence the first chapter. Chapter 2 highlights research and theories used in treatment programs and explores how these theories are utilized by evaluators. A key feature of Chapter 2 is the focus on mental health and substance use research, evidence, theories, and frameworks. We can no longer sit quietly and watch as injustices occur at every road in our evaluation journey. A key issue that evaluators must embrace and uphold is evidence that addiction is a disease. Despite mounds of evidence that addiction is in fact a disease that requires the same level of funding, care, support, and attention as any other disease, more than half of the US population does not believe that addiction is a brain disease. Moreover, individuals with this disease do not receive fair, equal, quality, or just treatment. Chapter 3 is all about evaluation methods used in treatment programs. This core chapter explores the basic steps of evaluation, evaluation designs, approaches, and theories. Chapter 4 highlights systems that support recovery. Treatment programs are located within a broader system.

These systems have significant impacts on how programs and activities work. Chapter 5 includes real-world examples of treatment program evaluations. Chapter 6 stresses the importance of a public health approach to the evaluation of treatment programs and what this looks like in treatment program settings. This chapter moves beyond the individualistic focus of clinical treatment into broader policy, social, and environmental domains. Chapter 7 summarizes key information from the text and highlights communication, hope, equity, and healing.

Pedagogical Features

Every chapter in this book begins with learning objectives, content, wrap-up, discussion questions, additional resources, and references. Critical public health messages for public health are bolded throughout this text as Public Health Takeaways. These highlight my perspectives about the evaluation of treatment programs in an authentic way. The appendix includes even more examples of resources that may support evaluators working in various settings.

1 Introduction and Overview

CONTENTS

DOI: 10.4324/9781003290728-1

Learning Objectives

After reading this chapter, you should be able to:

- Summarize the history of substance use in our world.
- Define mental health, mental illness, co-occurring disorders, substance use disorders, and prevalence at the United States and global level.
- Describe elements of a public health approach and the evaluation of programs that treat mental health and substance use disorders.
- Understand positionality and how it applies to the evaluation of treatment programs.

Orientation

Thinking about mental health, substance use, needs, evaluation—having everything in one chapter sometimes it feels like a lot to take in. As we begin this journey together, know that throughout this text, I use the term "We" because in my work, I never work alone. I might be talking with a team member about how to evaluate a medication-assisted treatment (MAT) program, interviewing a community member about recovery, or extracting clinical data from an electronic health record. In all these instances, I am more than just me. I am we. I live in the United States of America. Our approaches, research, and ideas about treatment programs might be different from a global perspective. I recognize this and write from my lived experiences, professional knowledge, and public health training. While I do not have the experiences of evaluating programs in Canada, Norway, or Japan … I know their programs, methods, and ideas offer something that we can all learn from. In this text, I add global perspectives and together we will explore some of the best ways to evaluate treatment programs. Together, we can contribute to the knowledge base of what makes treatment programs effective.

This text is for anyone who wants to know more about effective treatment programs. One of the statistics that I see first-hand in my life and in my work with treatment programs is that only 10.4% of individuals with a substance use disorder ever receive treatment (Substance Abuse and Mental Health Services Administration, 2019). Of this small percentage of individuals that actually receive treatment, just 33% receive evidence-based treatment, or treatment that is demonstrated effective by rigorous evaluation. Advocates, experts, researchers, evaluators, educators, providers, and communities are calling for a public health approach to address one of the greatest public health crises of our time, drug use, misuse, and related consequences.

A Public Health Approach

This book focuses on a public health approach toward the evaluation of treatment programs.

Public health is the science of preventing disease and injury and promoting and protecting the health of populations and communities (SAMHSA & Office of the Surgeon General, 2017). Public health approaches integrate multiple socioecological factors into the prevention efforts for the greatest population health impact. **Public health systems** involved in research, evaluation, treatment, and policy change include federal, state, local, and tribal agencies, non-profit organizations, for-profit organizations, community organizations, partners, and more.

A 2017 report from the US Surgeon General's Report on Alcohol, Drugs, and Health calls for change and a public health approach for addressing the factors that contribute to substance use disorders (SUD) in our nation (SAMHSA & Office of the Surgeon General, 2017). This report endorses a public health systems approach to substance misuse (prevention, treatment, and follow-up) including the following areas:

- Define problem through systematic collection of data.
- Identify risk and protective factors.
- Work across public and private sectors to create and test interventions that address SDOH.
- Support broad implementation of effective, evidence-based prevention, treatment, and recovery efforts.
- Monitor the impact of interventions (SAMHSA & Office of the Surgeon General, 2017).

As evaluators, public health advocates, social justice leaders, researchers, students, policy developers, and influencers, we want positive change. The first step in a public health approach is defining what the problem is and shared definitions. A public health approach requires us to consider what aspects of treatment programs and policy are not working, and change them. Throughout this text, we will use the following graphic to explore various aspects of treatment and evaluation.

By using Figure 1.1 as a guide, let's consider the following sections of the public health approach to evaluating treatment programs:

Understanding (steps 1–2)

- What is the problem? Situation analysis, surveillance, stakeholder perspectives, and observation.

Public Health Approach to Evaluating Substance Misuse Treatment Programs

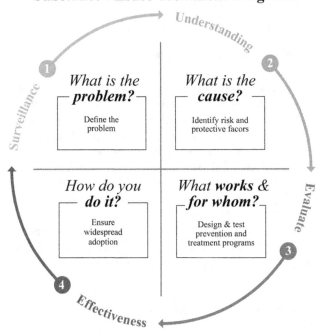

Figure 1.1 A Public Health Approach for the Evaluation of Treatment Programs.

- What is the cause? Identify risk and protective factors, acknowledge social justice issues, social determinants of health, socioecological factors at from the individual level to the chronosystem level.
- Which interventions work and for whom? Develop and test strategies and pilot studies; conduct formative research and research synthesis; and incorporate stakeholder perspectives. Do not continue interventions or policy that are ineffective or, in some cases, do more harm than good.
- How do you do the work? Consider the needs, resources, and context.

Evaluating (step 3)

- What are we doing? Activities, interventions, process monitoring, evaluation, and quality assessments.
- Are we doing what we said we would do? Outputs and indicators show us what programs are doing.

Effectiveness (step 4)

- Are interventions effective? Outcome evaluations can tell us about effectiveness.
- Is there widespread adoption of interventions, programs, and policies? Survey and surveillance activities help document adoption of activities and effectiveness.

This chapter focuses on understanding or answering the question, "What is the problem?" (step 1). We answer this question through surveillance efforts, program reports, national surveys, and data at the local, community, state, nation, and global level. Throughout the text, you will learn how to frame the evaluation of substance use programs from a public health lens. By using Figure 1.1 as a guide, the sections in this text include mentions of step 1 to illustrate the process.

First, let's consider your own definitions of the terms that we will be using in this book.

- Public health is _____.
- Public health systems are _____.
- Mental health is _____.
- Mental illness is _____.
- Substance use is _____.
- Substance misuse is _____.
- Co-occurring disorders are _____.
- Recovery means _____.

As a researcher and evaluator, I automatically want to know how all readers define these terms.

However, that is impossible, so let's consider some commonly used definitions for these terms.

- Mental health refers to an individual's well-being and state of mind.
- Mental illness refers to something that impacts an individual's mental state and how they think, feel, communicate, and behave.
- Substance use refers to the use of alcohol or other drugs (illegal or legal).
- Substance misuse and abuse is a pattern of harmful consumption of substances for mind-altering purposes.
- Co-occurring disorders refer to the co-occurrence of a psychoactive substance use disorder and another psychiatric disorder in the same individual.
- Recovery is an outcome or state of being that can be clinical or personal.

In writing this book, there was a pull to include mental health, mental illness, substance use, substance abuse, substance abuse disorder, substance misuse, alcohol use disorder (AUD), addiction, and drug use. Therefore, much of the treatment and treatment program evaluation blend multiple disciplines and bodies of research. To acknowledge a collective body of research, ideas, concepts, or meaning, I use the term mental health substance use disorder (MHSUD) to represent both disciplines and areas of treatment. The term mental health substance use (MHSU) is used to represent, a collection of ideas, or the overall concept of both MHSU without the clinical term disorder included. When I write *treatment program*, this may include a recovery program, a behavioral health program, an addiction treatment program, or various treatment programs that may be evaluated. *Other terms* used in this text will be described in various chapters, generally noted by bolded text.

Definitions Matter: Substances and Substance Use Disorder

In this text, when we use the term "substance," it means any psychoactive compound that has the potential to cause health and social problems, including addiction. Substances may be legal like alcohol or tobacco, or illegal like heroin and cocaine. Some substances are prescribed for medical purposes, like hydrocodone or oxycodone (e.g., Oxycontin, Vicodin, and Lortab). These substances are often categorized based on their pharmacological and behavioral effects (McLellan, 2017).

- Nicotine—cigarettes, vapor-cigarettes, cigars, chewing tobacco, and snuff
- Alcohol—including all forms of beer, wine, and distilled liquors
- Cannabinoids—marijuana, hashish, hash oil, and edible cannabinoids
- Opioids—heroin, methadone, buprenorphine, oxycodone, Vicodin, and Lortab
- Depressants—benzodiazepines (e.g., Valium, Librium, and Xanax) and Barbiturates (e.g., Seconal)
- Stimulants—cocaine, amphetamine, methamphetamine, methylphenidate (e.g., Ritalin), and atomoxetine (e.g., Stratera)
- Hallucinogens—LSD, mescaline, and MDMA (e.g., Ecstasy)

Substance Use Disorders (SUD)

The beginnings of substance use can be traced back to 7,000–5,000BC when archaeological findings suggested that alcoholic beverages were consumed by humans. Human use of poppy plants and hemp fibers began more than 6,000 years ago (Escohotado, 1999). More recently, Mann and colleagues reported on the last 100 years of alcoholism and describe alcohol consumption and disease characteristics (Mann, 2000). The National Academies of Science and researchers summarized the last 150 years of alcoholism in the United States in their report, *Alcohol in America: Taking Action to Prevent Abuse* (Olson & Gerstein, 1985). Jensen and colleagues report on the timeline and impacts of criminalizing addiction in the United States, this will be discussed more in

Chapter 6 (Jensen et al., 2004). The following timeline summarizes milestones in the history of alcoholism from these three previous publications.

Box 1.1   History of Alcoholism and Addiction and Key Milestones

1700s—Colonists of North America view heavy drinking as normal, distilled, and fermented liquors considered essential.

1784—Benjamin Rush describes the overwhelming and irresistible desire to consume alcohol.

1813—Pearson and Sutton describe delirium tremens.

1800s—Concept of addiction emerges, temperance movement gains support. US and European countries address excessive alcohol consumption which disproportionately impacted working class families during industrialization.

1835—Alexis deTocqueville reports 1.5 million of America's 13 million citizens vow to never consume alcohol again.

1880s—Degenerationism emerges as a medical explanation for social problems caused by excessive alcohol consumption where acquired character traits passed on to offspring resulted in different symptoms and diseases such as impulsivity, alcoholism, stroke, or dementia.

1900s—Anti-Saloon League follows temperance movement, 18th Amendment ratified, Alcohol Prohibition enforced 1919 to 1933.

1920s—Bootlegging, moonshining, speakeasies thrive during the Prohibition era.

1933—Roosevelt repeals Prohibition through the 21st Amendment.

1934—Germany requires sterilization of individuals with physical and mental disabilities, including severe alcoholism, Nazi regime murders unknown number of alcohol-dependent patients.

1930s—Alcoholics Anonymous (AA) created and shows support for individuals with addiction.

1942—Jellinek's article posits that alcoholism is a disease not a moral failing.

1954—World Health Organization agrees with Jellinek's disease model.

1955—Symptoms of alcohol withdrawal noted by Victor and Adams.

1960—Jellinek publishes the Disease Concept of Alcoholism, outlining adaption of cell metabolism, tolerance, and withdrawal symptoms as the core challenges with alcoholism.

1967—Feuerlein promotes modern disease concept of alcoholism, calling for equal rights and medical treatment for alcohol-dependent patients.

1968—German courts confirm full insurance coverage of alcoholism-related medical treatment costs.

1971—National Institute on Alcohol Abuse and Alcoholism formed as part of the Alcohol, Drug Abuse, and Mental Health Administration.

1972—First national evaluation of treatment effectiveness (Drug Abuse Reporting Program), post-treatment follow-up outcome studies begin in the United States.

1980s—NIDA conducts large-scale evaluation and treatment outcome prospective study (TOPS) building evidence that treatment for drug addiction is effective.

1984—Legal drinking age in United States was raised from 18 to 21 years.

1986—Anti-Drug Abuse Act signed by President Nixon increases the number of drug offenses with mandatory minimum sentences; US prison population rapidly increases.

2001—US state prison population increases to 316%.

(Source: Jensen et al., 2004; Mann, 2000; Olson and Gerstein, 1985)

While beyond the scope of this text, we know from this history and current research that the etiology of SUD involves genetic, neurobiological, psycho-pharmacological, personality-related, and environmental factors (Sher et al., 1996). Check out the resource sections at the end of each chapter for more information about SUD.

Public Health Take Away—More than 20 million Americans over age 12 are impacted by SUD (National Center for Drug Abuse Statistics, 2021). SUD is a significant public health problem (step 1).

Diagnosing Substance Use Disorder

Most people who use drugs do not become addicted to them (Volkow et al., 2017). What contributes to differences in addiction status is an individual's susceptibility based on genetic, environmental, and developmental factors that are largely out of a person's control. Researchers have found that individuals are more likely to develop SUD if they have a family history, early exposure to drug use, exposure to high risk environments, and certain mental illnesses (Stanis & Andersen, 2014; Volkow et al., 2016, 2017).

The American Psychiatric Association (APA) maintains the *Diagnostic and Statistical Manual of Mental Disorders (DSM-5)* (American Psychiatric Association, 2013). Diagnosis involves physical exam, lab tests, and psychological evaluation. The *DSM-5* recognizes SUD resulting from the use of ten separate classes of drugs: alcohol; caffeine; cannabis; hallucinogens (phencyclidine or similarly acting arylcyclohexylamines, and other hallucinogens, such as LSD); inhalants; opioids; sedatives, hypnotics, or anxiolytics; stimulants (including amphetamine-type substances, cocaine, and other stimulants); tobacco; and other or unknown substances. Importantly, diagnosis is the driver for insurance payment, treatment, and levels of care. Criteria for SUD includes the following:

- Taking the substance in larger amounts or for longer than you're meant to.
- Wanting to cut down or stop using the substance but not managing to.
- Spending a lot of time getting, using, or recovering from use of the substance.
- Cravings and urges to use the substance.
- Not managing to do what you should at work, home, or school because of substance use.
- Continuing to use, even when it causes problems in relationships.
- Giving up important social, occupational, or recreational activities because of substance use.
- Using substances repeatedly, even when it puts you in danger.
- Continuing to use, even when you know you have a physical or psychological problem that could have been caused or made worse by the substance.
- Needing more of the substance to get the effect you want (tolerance).
- Development of withdrawal symptoms, which can be relieved by taking more of the substance (American Psychiatric Association, 2013).

The *DSM-5* allows clinicians to determine the severity of the SUD problem based on the number of symptoms identified. SUD is defined in the *DSM-5* as a maladaptive pattern of use characterized by two (or more) of 11 symptoms listed earlier (Martin et al., 2011). Two or three symptoms indicate a mild substance use disorder; four or five symptoms indicate a moderate substance use disorder, and six or more symptoms indicate a severe substance use disorder. Other options for clinicians when diagnosing a SUD include "in early remission," "in sustained remission," "on maintenance therapy" for certain substances, and "in a controlled environment" (American Psychiatric Association, 2013).

Alcohol Use Disorder (AUD)

Alcohol use disorder (AUD) include physical and behavioral impacts like withdrawal, tolerance, and cravings (Schick et al., 2020). About 5% of the population in the United States has been diagnosed with an AUD. Gender differences with AUD are notable, where globally, males report higher rates of AUD than females (7.8% for males vs. 1.5% for females) (American Psychiatric Association, 2013). While males are more likely to be diagnosed with an AUD, females experience greater negative consequences because of their AUD (NSDUH, Substance Abuse and Mental Health Services Administration, 2019). Differences in racial/ethnic prevalence of AUD have also been noted. The highest rate of AUD is among American Indian and Alaska Native populations, with 19.2% of the population reporting AUD. Black and African American populations report 14.4% AUD followed by Whites at 14.0%, Hispanics at 13.6%, and Asian American and Pacific Islanders at 10.6% (Vaeth et al., 2017).

Public Health Takeaway—Of the 15 million individuals in American with an AUD, less than 8.0% receive treatment (National Center for Drug Abuse

Statistics, 2021). AUD impacts American Indian and Alaska Native populations the most. A public health perspective requires us to determine *why* individuals with AUD do not receive treatment (step 2) and why American Indian and Alaska Native populations are differentially impacted.

Mental Illness (MI)

Mental illness (MI) and mental health (MH) are terms that we will use throughout this text to describe participant and treatment program characteristics. One distinguishing characteristic of a MI is that symptoms generally do not resolve without treatment.

According to the National Survey on Drug Use and Health [NSDUH], the percentage of adults who had any mental illness (AMI) in the past year increased from 17.7% (or 39.8 million people) in 2008 to 20.6% (or 51.5 million people) in 2019 (NSDUH, 2018). Over that same period, the percentage who had serious mental illness (SMI) in the past year increased from 3.7% (or 8.3 million people) to 5.2% (or 13.1 million people) (NSDUH, 2018).

Mental health is about our psychological and emotional wellbeing. An individual's mental health history is often considered within a treatment context. There are diverse ways that mental health is discussed in our work. Sometimes concepts are explored from a body and mind perspective, where physical health relates to the absence of disease and mental health refers to how we think, behave, and feel. The intersection of mental and physical health must be acknowledged because we must have both to experience optimum health.

Co-Occurring Mental Health Issues and SUD

A word on the term co-occurring, also called dual diagnosis, concurrent, and comorbidity, refers to the presence of more than one MHSUD that occur at the same time, and require treatment (Hakobyan et al., 2020). This phenomenon is described differently based on where you live and what clinical practices that are followed. For example, the World Health Organization [WHO] and many countries in the United Kingdom use the term *dual diagnosis*. Canadians use the term concurrent disorder. In the United States, we use the term co-occurring disorders. Australia and New Zealand use the terms coexisting MHSUDs.

Among adults aged 18 or older in 2019, 24.5% (or 61.2 million people) had either any mental illness (AMI) or an SUD in the past year, 16.8% (or 42.0 million people) had AMI but not an SUD, 3.9% (or 9.7 million people) had an SUD but not AMI, and 3.8% (or 9.5 million people) had both AMI and an SUD.

Public Health Takeaway—More than one in five adults over age 18 in the United States have an MI and 50% of people with SUD also experience MI (National Center for Drug Abuse Statistics, 2021). A public health approach requires comprehensive prevention, intervention, and treatment strategies that address the underlying causes or conditions that allow SUD and MI to persist (steps 2–3).

Recovery is a term frequently used in treatment programs and substance abuse literature that refers to an outcome or a state of being. The American Society of Addiction Medicine (ASAM) asserts that a patient is in recovery when they have reached a state of physical and psychological health such that their abstinence from dependency-producing drugs is complete and comfortable (ASAMa, n.d.). Clinicians view a person as being in recovery or not in recovery using objective ratings to assess status. In a clinical recovery setting, the definition of recovery does not vary between one person and the next (Slade & Wallace, 2017). For example, ASAM indicates that recovery from alcoholism is based on the following six areas: (1) sobriety, comfortable abstinence from alcohol, and/or other dependency-producing drugs, (2) improvement in aspects of physical health previously adversely affected by alcohol use, (3) improvement in family relationships and/or resolution of conflict in close relationships, (4) improvement in functional responsibilities and self-care, (5) progress toward resolution of related emotional difficulties, and (6) willingness to share recovery state with others (2005).

Personal definitions of recovery do not follow ASAM or clinical definitions. The subjective ways in which individuals define recovery is often based on a process that involves hope, identity, meaning, and personal responsibility (Slade & Wallace, 2017). The lack of shared definitions about recovery led researchers to develop a national project, "What is Recovery?" They surveyed 9,341 individuals throughout the United States to learn more about their definitions of recovery and how they changed over time (Kaskutas et al., 2014). Results from this research show that the following definitions of recovery received the highest levels of support:

- About 97% agreed that recovery is managing negative feelings without using drugs or drinking
- About 98% agreed that recovery is being honest with self and taking responsibility for the things they can change
- About 99% agreed that recovery is taking responsibility for the things they change and a process of growth and development (Kaskutas et al., 2014).

Data on recovery in the United States indicates that about 8.2% of adults in the country are in recovery from drug or alcohol problems and 12.5% of adults are in recovery from a mental health issue (NSDUH, 2018). The frequency of recovery varies based on age, where 4.8% of individuals aged 18 to 25 are in recovery from drug or alcohol use compared with 9.0% of adults aged 26 to 49 (NSDUH, 2018). In contrast, 17.4% of individuals aged 18 to 25 are in recovery from a mental health issue compared with 13.6% of adults aged 26 to 49 (NSDUH, 2018). Differences in recovery frequencies by age may be due to the development of alcohol and drug problems later in life, where younger age groups are less likely to experience recovery because they have not lived as long with the disease.

Public Health Takeaway—Only 8.2% of adults in the United States are in recovery (National Center for Drug Abuse Statistics, 2021). A public health approach requires professionals to consider what is happening to the other 92% of adults who are not in recovery (step 2). A fundamental message from the recovery community is that there are many paths to recovery, public health approaches to recovery address conditions, cultural values, and psychological needs, while promoting the four pillars of recovery (health, home, purpose, and community).

Substance Use Disorder Treatment

We know that only 10% of individuals with an SUD ever receive treatment (Substance Abuse and Mental Health Services Administration, 2019). Treatment statistics are summarized in the following text are based on the 2019 NSDUH report.

Treatment among people aged 12 or older in 2019, 1.5% (or 4.2 million people) received any substance use treatment in the past year, and 1.0% (or 2.6 million people) received substance use treatment at a specialty facility in the past year. Among people aged 12 or 19, 2.1 million received substance use treatment at a self-help group, 1.7 million received treatment at a rehabilitation facility as an outpatient, 1.3 million received treatment at a mental health center as an outpatient, 1.0 million received treatment at a rehabilitation facility as an inpatient, and 948,000 received treatment at a private doctor's office. Among the 21.6 million people aged 12 or older who needed substance use treatment from 2018 to 2019, 12.2% (or 2.6 million people) received substance use treatment at a specialty facility.

Reasons Why People Do Not Seek Treatment

Among the 18.9 million people aged 12 or older in 2019 with an SUD in the past year who did not receive treatment at a specialty facility, 95.7% (or 18.1 million people) did not feel that they needed treatment, 3.0% (or 577,000 people) felt that they needed treatment but did not try to get treatment, and 1.2% (or 236,000 people) felt that they needed treatment and tried to get treatment (NSDUH, Substance Abuse and Mental Health Services Administration, 2019).

Mental Health (MH) Services Data

Among adolescents aged 12 to 17, the percentage who received mental health services in a specialty mental health setting (inpatient or outpatient care) from 2018 to 2019 increased from 11.8% (or 2.9 million people) in 2002 to 16.7% (or 4.1 million people). Over that same period, the percentage who received mental health services in a general medical setting in the past year increased from 2.7% (or 657,000 people) to 3.7% (or 902,000 people). The percentage who received mental health services in an education setting in the past year increased from 12.1% (or 2.9 million people) in 2009 to 15.4% (or 3.7 million people) in 2019.

Among adults aged 18 or older, the percentage who received any mental health services from 2018 to 2019, increased from 13.0% (or 27.2 million people) in 2002 to 16.1% (or 40.2 million people) in 2019. Over that same time period, the percentage who received prescription medication for a mental health issue increased from 10.5% (or 22.0 million people) to 13.1% (or 32.6 million people), the percentage who received outpatient mental health services in the past year increased from 7.4% (or 15.5 million people) to 8.3% (or 20.6 million people), and the percentage who received inpatient mental health services in the past year increased slightly from 0.7% (or 1.5 million people) to 1.0% (or 2.4 million people). Among adults aged 18 or older with past year AMI, receipt of mental health services in the past year increased from 40.9% (or 16.2 million people) in 2008 to 44.8% (or 23.0 million people) in 2019. Among the 13.1 million adults aged 18 or older in 2019 with past year SMI, 65.5% (or 8.6 million people) received mental health services in the past year, which was similar to the percentage in each year from 2008 through 2018 (Substance Abuse and Mental Health Services Administration, 2019).

Public Health Takeaway—Only 10.0% of adults ever seek treatment and just 20% of individuals in drug treatment programs are women (National Center for Drug Abuse Statistics, 2021). A public health approach requires us to consider the risk and protective factors associated with seeking treatment and differences in treatment seeking behaviors based on gender status (step 2).

NSDUH data presented earlier provide a snapshot of MHSU prevalence in the United States and insight about treatment needs and the types of treatment people receive. NSDUH data tell us the number of people affected and the magnitude of the MHSU problem, but they fail to describe causes of the problem and strategies necessary to address the problem from a public health perspective.

Understanding SUD Treatment Programs and Services

There are many different types of SUD treatment programs and services in the United States. While we cannot review or even know every type of treatment program, we can look at examples and descriptions (California Health Care Foundation, 2018). Understanding the different types of treatment programs and services is essential for evaluators working in treatment settings (Table 1.1).

Treatment Program Levels of Care

Treatment programs provide individuals with a variety of resources and support that meet their unique needs. There are five levels of care when considering an individual's treatment needs. **Level 0.5** is the lowest level of care. This includes 15 hours of early intervention. Level 0.5 targets individuals who, for a known reason, are at risk of developing substance-related problems, or a service for those for whom there is not yet sufficient information to document a diagnosable substance use disorder. **Level 1.0** represents outpatient services and a minimum of 84 treatment hours completed. Level 1.0 may include recovery or

Table 1.1 SUD Treatment Programs and Services Example

	Description
Driving under the influence programs	Court-mandated educational sessions for individuals with DUI convictions
Emergency medical services	Hospital emergency services for people with SUD
Narcotic treatment programs	Replacement narcotic therapy to individuals with OUD
Outpatient SUD services	Outpatient medical facility provides variety of SUD services and non-medical SUD support
Residential medical services	Medical services in a residential setting for individuals with alcohol/drug related problems
Residential nonmedical services	Nonmedical care and recovery support services for adults in a residential setting, may include detoxification, group, individual, and education sessions, treatment or recovery planning

motivational enhancement therapies and strategies delivered in a variety of settings. Level 1.0 may also include a relapse prevention component. This could include group or individual sessions that address the individual's treatment needs. **Level 2.1** includes services address the needs of people with addiction and co-occurring conditions. Typically, 2.1 services are organized treatment times that may occur before or after school and work, or at other times throughout the day. **Level 2.5** provides 20 or more hours of service per week to address multidimensional instability. Typically created as an outpatient service or partial hospitalization approach, Level 2.5 provides intensive services for individuals who do not need to be hospitalized. **Level 3.1** includes low-intensity residential services with 24-hour support and structure from qualified staff. Level 3.1 usually includes 4 hours of clinical service per week. **Level 3.3** includes high intensity residential services for adults only. Trained counselors provider 24-hour care and medical staff are available. **Level 3.5** is clinically managed medium-intensity residential services for adolescents rather than adults. **Level 3.7** targets adolescents and adults who need to be medically monitored and required intensive inpatient services to address withdrawal symptoms. **Level 4.0** is medically managed intensive inpatient services for adolescents and adults. Level 4.0 includes 24-hour nursing care, medical staff, and provides support for individuals who have severe conditions or are considered unstable (ASAMb, n.d.). Figure 1.2 outlines the continuum of care provided by various treatment programs based on level of need.

More on Public Health Approaches, Treatment, and Evaluation

This text is unique because it calls for evaluation approaches that address the broader public health domains that may contribute to effective treatment. Earlier in this chapter, we reviewed a public health model (Figure 1.1) used to

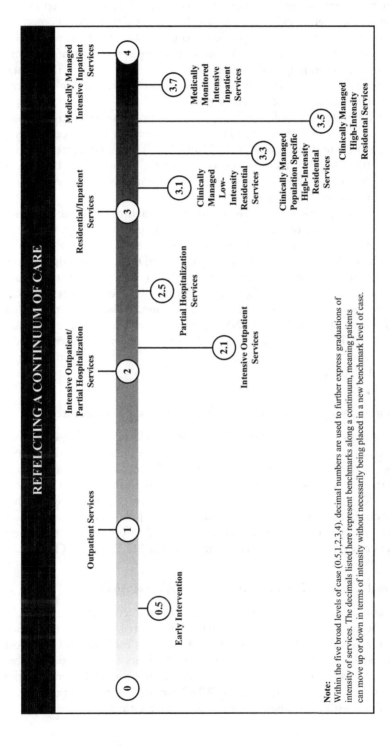

Figure 1.2 Treatment Program Continuum of Care.

evaluate treatment programs, beginning with defining the problem (step 1). We also reviewed key terms and definitions involved in a public health approach to evaluating treatment programs. This knowledge combined with public health paradigms used at various levels in the prevention, intervention, treatment, and follow-up process can help evaluators as they navigate a complex world of data, environmental, societal, and political factors that contribute to treatment program effectiveness, or lack of effectiveness.

Figure 1.3 outlines a public health approach to preventing opioid overdoses using three levels of prevention: (1) primary prevention, (2) secondary prevention, and (3) tertiary prevention (ASTHO, 2017). Treatment programs may utilize all three levels or focus on just one level. Evaluators should be familiar with these areas and know that some treatment program evaluations will include all levels, or, in some cases, just one.

Public health practice paradigms and the evaluation of treatment programs may be different based on the treatment focus, outcome, or context. Figure 1.3 demonstrates levels of prevention for opioid overdoses and opioid use disorder treatment. A note on acronyms used in Figure 1.3: **PDMP**s are prescription drug monitoring programs. **Ignition interlock** is a device that measures the blood-alcohol limit of a driver when they get into a car and prevents individuals from driving if the concentration is over a specified limit. **Naloxone** is medication used to reverse opioid overdose. **SNEP**s are syringe needle exchange programs (ASTHO, 2017). A public health approach to SUD results in a substantial cost savings to society. The next section outlines costs of treatment in the United States and globally.

The Costs of Drug and Alcohol Abuse Treatment in the United States

The costs of treatment vary. We know that when evidence-based interventions are utilized, the cost savings can be 58:1 or for every dollar spent, the savings exceeds $58 (SAMHSA & Office of the Surgeon General, 2017). However, a key issue with treatment and cost expenditures is that most treatment is not evidence-based. A 2016 study published by the Recovery Centers of America reports that the costs of treatment in the United States is $15.6 billion per year. The most expensive treatment costs are detoxification at $332.55 per day and the lowest treatment costs is outpatient methadone treatment at $17.57 per day (Table 1.2).

Social and Economic Costs Due to Drug and Alcohol Abuse

Few countries have established social and economic cost estimates for substance abuse. Among countries that have enumerated the economic costs, different methods, contextual factors, and data are used. Inconsistent cost methods make it difficult to accurately assess the costs to society on a global scale. What we know about global costs comes from a 2004 report by the World Health Organization (WHO). WHO reported costs by country, year, and total cost estimates. Their report found that US estimates were the highest

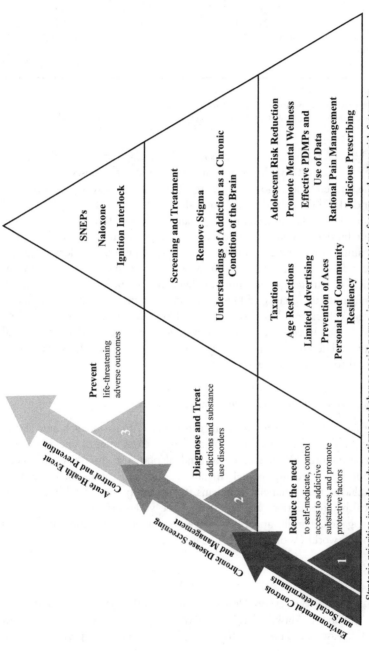

Figure 1.3 Public Health Paradigms, Treatment, and Evaluation of Opiates.

Strategic priorities include reduce stigma and change social norms, increase protective factors and reduce risk factors in communities, strengthen collaborations, improve prevention infrastructure, optimize the use of data for decision making.

Adapted from ASTHO, 2017

Table 1.2 Costs of Treatment for Substance Abuse in the United States, 2016

Treatment Type	Census[*]	Cost Per Day[**]	Cost Per Person	Total Cost
Detoxification	71,060	$332.55	$121,381.07	$ 8,625,338,797
Residential	102,934	$119.03	$43,446.04	$4,472,075,173
Outpatient	276,027	$19.78	$7,219.13	$1,992,675,157
Outpatient (Methadone)	431,780	$17.57	$6,414.47	$2,769,639,529
Total				$17,859,728,657

Notes
* Based on the average population per day of treatment centers.
** Costs per day adjusted for inflation(Source: Recovery Centers of America, 2017).

at $184.6 billion, followed by Japan $5.7 billion, Canada $7.52 billion, and Chile $2.69 billion (2018). More recent reports about the costs of substance abuse in the United States show that the total overall costs exceeds $420 billion annually and $120 billion health care costs alone (McLellan, 2017). The costs of drug and alcohol abuse are not just financial. We know that substance abuse places undue burdens on our health, education, employment, and social systems. Substance abuse is a significant public health problem and may lead to cardiovascular conditions, pregnancy complications, teenage pregnancy, human immunodeficiency virus/acquired immunodeficiency syndrome (HIV/AIDS), sexually transmitted diseases (STDs, domestic violence, child abuse, sexual abuse, motor vehicle crashes, homicide, and suicide (SAMHSA & Healthy People, n.d.). Other costs include lost productivity, increased crime-related costs, and overall decreased quality of life. We will review more about evaluation methods used to estimate costs in Chapters 3 and 5.

Global Race, Age, Place, and Socioeconomic Status

We know that MHSUD impacts every race, age, place, and socioeconomic status. The United States and Canada have some of the highest rates of suicide (World Health Organization, 2019). Depression and alcohol use disorders have been linked to suicide, especially in high income countries. Reasons for these associations include crisis, financial problems, relationships, and health problems (World Health Organization, 2019). Alcohol use varies across the globe where Germany, Uganda, Latvia, and Spain have the highest consumption patterns reported in the world (World Health Organization, 2018).

Race

The 2018 National Survey on Drug Use and Health [NSDUH] reports that American Indian or Alaska Native (AI/AN) populations report the highest rates of SUD. Based on data for individuals 12 and older, SUD prevalence data are as follows, 10.5% AIANs, 9.3% Native Hawaiian or Other Pacific Islander, 7.7% White, 7.1% Hispanic or Latino, 6.9% Black or African American, and 4.8% Asian American (2019). These rates are similar to Vaeth and colleague's publication on the prevalence of AUD (2017).

Public Health Takeaway—When considering the role of race and SUD, it is essential to consider the underlying causes that contribute to higher rates of disease. For example, many minority and underserved populations experience challenges when accessing care such as transportation, financial considerations, discrimination, stigma, language barriers, or cultural differences (step 3).

Sex, Gender, and Special Populations

Sex and gender roles matter when it comes to understanding the prevalence and treatment of MHSUD. Sex refers to one's physiological structures and sex assigned at birth as male, female, or intersex (Gilbert et al., 2018). While beyond the scope of this text, evaluators and researchers must be cognizant of how physical sex is defined within a study population. Gender is a social construct that includes how we feel, act, behave, see the world, and interact with others (Grant et al., 2015). AUD, SUD, and MH disorders vary by gender, for example, men are more likely to be diagnosed with AUD than women (Schick et al., 2020). Research on gender minority populations, which include transgender, gender non-binary, gender queer, and other gender non-conforming groups, has found that binge drinking is higher among transgender populations, especially in early adulthood (Schuler et al., 2018). Consequences related to AUD are more common and more severe among gender minority populations, for example stigma, discrimination, and negative attitudes about gender identity have been linked to transgender-related issues (Gilbert et al., 2018). We also know that women are twice as likely as men to be diagnosed with a MI (Nochaiwong et al., 2021). Other special population subgroups that experience higher rates of MHSUD include homeless individuals, prisoners, veterans, and sex workers (Aldridge et al., 2018).

Age

An individual's age when they first use a substance is associated with increased risk for problematic substance use and SUD (Richmond-Rakerd et al., 2017). Most individuals with a SUD started using before they were 18 and developed a disorder by age 20 (Dennis et al., 2002). Researchers have found that 15.2% of people who begin drinking before the age of 14 will develop alcohol abuse or dependence. In contrast, just 2.1% of individuals that wait until they are 21 or older to begin drinking will develop alcohol abuse or dependence (Richmond-Rakerd et al., 2017). The rate is higher for prescription drug use where 25% of individuals who begin abusing before age 13 will develop a SUD in their lifetime. Marijuana is the most common substance used in early adolescence and 13% of individuals with a SUD began using marijuana before they were 14

(Dennis et al., 2002). Previous researchers report differences in substance use patterns based on age and race. For example, African American individuals initiate alcohol use at older ages and engage in less under-age drinking than Whites (Zapolski et al., 2014).

Public Health Takeaway—Prevention of substance use must begin early and target groups most at risk for SUD. Marijuana is the most common substance used in early adolescence, implementing environmental controls, and addressing social determinants while promoting protective factors is an essential step in the prevention early intervention process (see Figure 1.3).

Trauma

When we think about MHSUDs, it is easy to just look at the disease, rates, deaths, and risk factors. However, we must stop to consider the cause. MHSUD is often the symptom or result of unresolved trauma. Exposure to trauma, especially during childhood is associated with SUD and PTSD. Researchers have found that childhood trauma impacts neural structure and functioning. Later in life this can lead to cognitive deficits, schizophrenia, depression, bipolar disorder, PTSD, and SUD (Khoury et al., 2010). Research from a national survey of youth reports that those who experienced physical abuse or sexual abuse and assault were at least three times more likely to report abusing substances compared to other youth without trauma histories (Funk et al., 2003). Researchers found that 70% of youth receiving treatment for SUD had a history of trauma (Khoury et al., 2010).

Place

Where we live impacts how we live and our overall health, including AUD, SUD, and MH.

Housing stress, which includes affordability, quality, stability, and loss of housing, is related to MHSUD. Researchers have studied the causal pathways using the social causation hypothesis as a guide, where stress related to living in poverty often contributes to psychopathology related to MHSUD behaviors and problems (Austin et al., 2021; Polcin et al., 2010).

Rural communities in the US report higher rates of SUD than more urban communities. Researchers report that rural counties have opioid prescribing rates and more deaths related to opioid overdoses. Social and environmental factors in rural locations may explain differences in prevalence rates. For example, the normalization of prescription opioid use in rural communities increases use and overdose rates. Isolation, lack of treatment facilities, social and cultural norms, and stigma that may be associated with seeking treatment (such as medication assisted treatment) are common (Bolinski et al., 2019).

We know that **low-income to middle-income countries** (LMIC) carry a disproportionate burden of MHSUDs. Higher prevalence in LMIC may be related to a lack of access to evidence-based prevention and treatment strategies.

A systematic review of LMICs reported that prisoners in these countries reported higher prevalence of MHSUD than general populations, where the prevalence of psychosis was 6.2%, 16.0% depression, 3.8% AUD, and 5.1% drug use disorders (Baranyi et al., 2019).

Lower Education and Unemployment

Education and employment are strong predictors of MHSUD. Previous research indicates that the level of education achieved is directly linked to depression prevalence, where higher levels of education are associated with lower levels of depression (Henkel, 2011). Similarly, employment status has been linked to depression, where individuals who are employed are less likely to be depressed than individuals who are not employed (Ritchie & Roser, 2018). Employment is also related to SUD where research has found that unemployment is significantly related to SU and development of SUD (Henkel, 2011). An emerging body of research indicates that educational attainment, economic conditions, and SUD are related, and countercyclical. While beyond the scope of this text, researchers documented the relationship between economic conditions, and factors like health insurance coverage, quality health care, risky health behaviors, poor diets, and drug and alcohol consumption patterns. Yet, most research available on socioeconomic conditions and SUD is focused on alcohol and not illicit drugs (Christopher et al., 2017).

Socioeconomic Status

Socioeconomic status (SES) has profound impacts on overall health and MHSUD prevalence. SES is thought to impact MHSUD prevalence by lifestyle choices. Although research is mixed, SES is related to lifestyle choices and these choices often explain physical health and psychological health (Wang & Geng, 2019). Individuals with lower SES are more likely to die from alcohol-related deaths than individuals with higher SES. One study found that individuals with low SES were two to five times more likely to die from alcohol-related deaths than individuals with high SES (Probst et al., 2020). This is somewhat of a paradox since individuals with lower SES report less alcohol consumption than higher SES groups (Lewer et al., 2016). One possible explanation for increased mortality in low SES groups is the addition of other risk factors like obesity, smoking, and other health conditions (Lewer et al., 2016; Probst et al., 2020).

Global Efforts to Address MHSUD

The United Nation's 2030 agenda for sustainable development includes a focus on reducing the harmful effects of alcohol and promoting mental health and well-being. The United Nations developed 17 Sustainable Development Goals (SDGs) with 169 targets from all UN member states in 2015. All member states agreed to achieve these goals, or at least try to by 2030. UN's target 3.4 relates to mental health and wellbeing, "By 2030, reduce one third premature mortality from noncommunicable diseases through prevention and treatment and promote mental health well-being." This SDG is supported by Indicator 3.4.2, which includes reducing the suicide mortality rate. UN's SDG target 3.5 relates to SUD, "Strengthen the prevention and treatment of substance use, including narcotic drug abuse and harmful use of alcohol" (World Health Organization, 2018). SDG Target 3.5 is supported by two indicators, 3.5.1, "Coverage of treatment interventions for SUD" and 3.5.2, "Harmful use of alcohol, defined according to the national context as alcohol per capita consumption within a calendar year in liters of pure alcohol" (World Health Organization, 2018).

Public Health Takeaway—Unfortunately, current global trends indicate that mental health problems and alcohol-related mortality and morbidity are increasing in the world, and impacts are greater and more pervasive across populations, constituting a public health crisis (steps 1–4).

Global Prevalence and Unmet Needs: Prevalence of MI/MH, SUD, and Comorbid Conditions

We know that one in ten people globally live with a mental health disorder (Ritchie & Roser, 2018). MI and MH disorders are under-reported and the complexities of estimating global prevalence of MI/MH disorders have been noted by previous researchers. What we know about the prevalence of MI/MH comes from the imputation of medical, epidemiological, and clinical data. The Global Burden of Disease study summarizes SUD with MHDs. The table and maps discussed later summarizes the disorder type, global population with the disorder based, differences across countries, the number of people with the disorder, and differences based on gender. (Table 1.3) (Map 1.1).

MHSUD Trends COVID-19

Our world continues to experience the global COVID-19 pandemic. As I type this chapter, the Delta variant is taking hold of communities, hospitals, and minds. Experts tell us that many of the impacts of COVID-19 on persons with MHSUD are indirect and difficult to measure (Volkow, 2020). For example, individuals may be deprioritized in clinical settings, experience greater isolation and stress, or not be able to access medications and treatments required for their recovery (Marel et al., 2021). Research, data sets, and findings are being published every day. The trends reported here are estimates based on the data available at the time this book was developed, this is what we know about COVID-10 impacts and MHSUD.

COVID-19 Populations at Risk and Health Problems

Researchers report that children, teens, elders, people with disabilities, and health workers are most at risk for MHSUD impacts due to the COVID-19

Table 1.3 Global Disorders, Country Differences, and Gender Differences, 2017

Disorder	Share of Global Population With Disorder (2017) [Difference across Countries]	Number of People with the Disorder (2017)	Share of Males: Females with Disorder (2017)
Any mental health disorder	10.7%	792 million	9.3% males 11.9% females
Depression	3.4% [2–6%]	264 million	2.7% males 4.1% females
Anxiety disorders	3.8% [2.5–7%]	284 million	2.8% males 4.7% females
Bipolar disorder	0.6% [0.3–1.2%]	46 million	0.55% males 0.65% females
Eating disorders (clinical anorexia & bulimia)	0.2% [0.1–1%]	16 million	0.13% males 0.29% females
Schizophrenia	0.3% [0.2–0.4%]	20 million	0.26% males 0.25% females
Any mental or substance use disorder	13% [11–18%]	970 million	12.6% males 13.3% females
Alcohol use disorder	1.4% [0.5–5%]	107 million	2% males 0.8% females
Drug use disorder (excluding alcohol)	0.9% [0.4–3.5%]	71 million	1.3% males 0.6% females

(Source: Ritchie & Roser, 2018).

pandemic (Javed et al., 2020). Health problems such as stress, anxiety, depressive symptoms, denial, anger, and fear have been noted by researchers across the globe (Torales et al., 2020). Researchers at Columbia University report increases in the global prevalence of mental health issues such as depression and anxiety during the COVID-19 pandemic (Castaldelli-Maia et al., 2021). However, in LMICs lower- and COVID-19 impacts are even more pronounced. One of the most notable findings from research is that LMIC countries had very limited access to MHSUD services before the pandemic. Resources that were available for individuals prior to the pandemic have been redirected to the COVID-19 response.

Although we will not cover every country in the world, here are some global MHSU trends. A nationwide study of 10,000 people in Bangladesh during the pandemic found a 33.0% prevalence of depression and 5% prevalence of suicide ideation (Mamun et al., 2021). In the United States, MHSU impacts are increasing. Throughout the pandemic 30% of adults in the US reported symptoms of anxiety and/or depressive disorder (Marel et al., 2021) and prior to the pandemic the percentage was 19%. We know that 20.0% of school-aged children have experienced worsened mental or emotional health since the

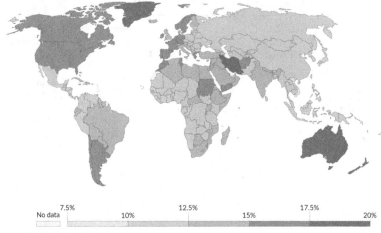

Share of population with mental health and substance use disorders, 2017

Share of population with any mental health or substance use disorder; this includes depression, anxiety, bipolar, eating disorders, alcohol or drug use disorders, and schizophrenia. Due to the widespread under-diagnosis, these estimates use a combination of sources, including medical and national records, epidemiological data, survey data, and meta-regression models.

Source: IHME, Global Burden of Disease   CC BY

Map 1.1 Share of Population with Mental Health and Substance Disorders, 2017. (Source: Ritchie & Roser, 2018).

pandemic began. Of the adults with symptoms of anxiety and/or depressive disorder during the pandemic, 20% felt they needed treatment but did not receive it (Marel et al., 2021). Deaths due to drug overdose increased during the pandemic, primarily driven by synthetic opioid use. In the United States, in the 12-month period ending in September 2020, there were 27.4 deaths due to drug overdose per 100,000, up from 21.3 per 100,000 in 2019. A recent study found that the combined prevalence of current depression, initiating or increasing substance use, and suicidal thoughts/ideation among US adults over 18 increased during the pandemic, where 28.6% reported depression, 18.2% reported initiating or increasing substance use, and 8.4% reported suicidal thoughts/ideation (McKnight-Eily et al., 2021).

Public Health Takeaway—Impacts of the COVID-19 pandemic on individuals and public health systems is clear. Evidence-based interventions are warranted to address conditions that place people at risk for MHSUD. Policy makers and advocates must consider how to increase treatment access while creating opportunities for community, connection, and support (steps 2–3).

Evaluation of Programs and Treatment Methods

This book will show you how to evaluate treatment programs using a public health approach. Evaluating treatment programs requires skill, understanding, humility, and recovery. If you or someone that you love has struggled with MHSUD, then you know it is essential to find programs that are effective. As evaluators, public health professionals, and recovery advocates our shared mission is to help individuals, families, and communities recover. We all want to know what works and what does not work. It is time to explore the role of evaluators in addressing the MHSUD crisis occurring in our world. We have the knowledge and the skills to find what works.

Our Position as Evaluators

If you have worked as an evaluator for a while, people usually have two responses or thoughts about evaluators. The first response, is generally something like ... "Oh, I better be on my best behavior, you have power to take away funding or write a bad report about my work." The second response, is, "What does it mean to be an evaluator?" Both responses demonstrate to me that evaluators have work to do. We must be acutely aware of our position, our bias, our approaches, our ethics, and our standards. We will cover this more in Chapter 3 and beyond. The American Evaluation Association (AEA) urges us to consider our positionality, meaning our individual identity (race, gender, sex, and age), our lived experiences social and historical movements, and how these change overtime (Alcoff, 1998). Evaluators must practice reflexivity, which requires us to consider our own bias and how this impacts our position within a given evaluation (van Draanen, 2017). Topics like ethics, professional standards, credentials, and power are inherent to any evaluation, but especially the evaluation of treatment programs.

When we think about treatment programs, our position and personal experiences impact how we interpret the events happening around us. We must be okay talking and thinking about our own recovery and our own brokenness. Here are some reflections to get you thinking about positionality, bias, and ethics. The cardiac surgeon conducting open-heart surgery cannot wait for the surgery to be over ... he needs to smoke a cigarette. The licensed addiction counselor drinks at the bar because she can find no other way to cope with the stories, the people, the stress. The social worker lives in a home where he experiences domestic violence, he does not leave. The evaluator cannot wait to drink the entire bottle of red wine after work. The family reunification advocate has not spoken to their children in 10 years. The law enforcement officer drinks too much at the bar and drives home. I write these reflections because they represent people who are living in two worlds. One of my elders explained this to me by saying that we are pitiful people, and we are star people. There is a dichotomy here that we must recognize. We will not always be star people, things will come up, we will lose our sense of balance and self-regulation, we might lash out, behave badly, or just not respond in ways that are honoring to others. Evaluators are human, so we live in these two worlds, and we must uphold certain standards, ethics, and positions.

My Position

I have worked in public health for almost two decades. Overall, I am healthy, no major complaints. I have been a social drinker for most of my adult years. I have never been diagnosed with an SUD, AUD, or MI. I do not drink alcohol anymore … . My time away from alcohol has given me perspectives about recovery that I did not think were possible. I wrote this a few months ago, it describes my thoughts about addiction and recovery.

Recovery is just like getting back on a bike, after a long sabbatical away from the roads. If we agree that recovery is about regaining what has been lost, today I got back on my road bike after a 5-year sabbatical. I know the benefits of riding, the serotonin and dopamine that are released with each mile, but I have had better excuses, why I should not ride. Some of these are based out of real fear, others denial.

- I will get hit by a semi and die on the road.
- I will get a flat tire in an area with no reception and be forced to walk with my bike on the tiny shoulder of the road, into a town with reception.
- I will not be able to get my shoes out of the locks on the pedals … this will result in the most gnarly crash one has ever seen.
- I will forget how to ride.

I am turning 45 in just a few days. I want to start regaining what I have lost. I got back on my bike. This is what happened. I thought the gears were missing, they were nowhere to be found … I figured it out, they were hidden just next to handlebars. I did not experience the most gnarly crash in history despite not being able to get my shoes out of the pedal locks. I rode for an hour … just 10 miles … through Camp Polk Meadows and Indian Ford Road. I was out of breath, thought I might have a massive heart attack, but I survived. Fear can paralyze you to do nothing, you never get back on the bike, you never try to stop drinking, you never end the unhealthy relationship, you don't say what needs to be said, you will not forgive others, you get the idea.

Early in recovery you get some speed, you figure out the gears, the safe roads, and places to be, these are the places that become your new normal. You see other people riding their bikes up hills, slow, struggling, some turning around, the hill is too high, recovery is too hard, the gears will not shift, the tires are flat, the semis are coming. Road bike model superstars, triathletes pass you on the road at about 100 mph. A feeling of unworthiness, not enough, lame, whale on the toothpick comes into the mind … sometimes this is how you will feel in recovery, listening to people that have the 39 years of sobriety and you have just two days … but this feeling will pass. The veil is lifted. You can see things on the bike that you would never see without recovery. The chipmunk standing bravely on the log. The Three Sisters mountains in all of their splendor. The man with his dog, walking through the meadow with the white Subaru that has been parked there forever. Patience in a man gripping binoculars with his head tilted up. The grace and kindness of cars and semis passing, giving you the space to fully recover, regain, get back the road that has been lost (Kelley, 2021).

Some describe being in recovery as having a veil lifted, a spiritual transformation of sorts, a new focus and clarity in thinking that was never possible in a drug-induced, hungover state of being. I agree with these descriptions because I have experienced them. I believe that we cannot work in treatment programs, with people, communities, families, systems if we are not in a recovery space ourselves, part of the **recovery generation**. If the opposite of treatment is recovery and recovery is about reigning what has been lost. What is it that you have lost? Sobriety. Self-regulation. Healthy relationships. Forgiveness. Time. Acceptance. Health. There are reciprocal benefits for evaluators working in treatment program settings. We learn about recovery and healing without having to be admitted, referred, or accepted. This is the ultimate payment and gift (Kelley, 2021).

Wrap-Up

We covered a ton of ground in this first chapter. You might be setting down the book and thinking, "No way." I am not going to read another page. Or you might be so engaged with the information and public health approach that you are now perusing the publicly available datasets located in the resource section of this chapter. Wherever you are at as we close this first chapter, know that a public health approach always begins with understanding and documenting the need, prevalence, or problem. If we don't document where we are at, we will never know where we need to be. What do you know about the evaluation of treatment programs now that you did not know before you started reading this chapter? What about your position as an evaluator? Have you considered your own bias, ethics, and professional standards? What do you think about your rightful place in the recovery generation? Now is the time. If you want to uncover more about how your lived experiences contribute to bias, check out the resources section at the end of this chapter and take Harvard's Project Implicit Bias test. The results may just surprise you.

Discussion Questions

1. What did you learn about the history of alcoholism as a disease from this chapter? How might this history influence your work as an evaluator?
2. What are the differences between mental health, mental illness, and substance use disorder? How might evaluators work with treatment programs to ensure interventions target specific treatment needs?
3. When you think about a public health approach to the evaluation of treatment programs, how does this differ from other evaluation approaches that are not informed from a public health perspective?

Additional Resources

Levels of Care and Policy

American Society of Addiction Medicine Continuum (ASAM) Levels of Care and Criteria, https://www.asamcontinuum.org/

American Society of Addiction Medicine Public Policy Statement, https://www.asam.org/advocacy/find-a-policy-statement

Screening tools

Mental Health America (MHA), Bipolar Disorder Screening Tool, https://screening.mhanational.org/bipolar/

National Institute of Drug Abuse (NIDA), How to Recognize a Substance Use Disorder, https://www.drugabuse.gov/publications/step-by-step-guides-to-finding-treatment-drug-use-disorders/if-you-have-problem-drugs-adults/how-to-recognize-substance-use-disorder

Harvard's Project Implicit Bias, https://implicit.harvard.edu/implicit/takeatest.html

Addiction Technology Transfer Center Network Anti-Stigma Toolkit, https://attcnetwork.org/sites/default/files/2019-04/Anti-Stigma%20Toolkit.pdf

Treatment Centers

Find Treatment Centers Near You, https://findtreatment.gov/

Substance Abuse and Mental Health Services Administration (SAMHSA) Behavioral Health Treatment Centers, https://findtreatment.samhsa.gov/

Public datasets

Our World in Data: https://ourworldindata.org/

2019 National Survey on Drug use and Health (NSDUH) Annual National Report, https://www.samhsa.gov/data/report/2019-nsduh-annual-national-report

Kaiser Family Foundation Mental Health and Substance Use Indicators and Trends, https://www.kff.org/state-category/mental-health/alcohol-drug-dependence-and-abuse/

References

American Society of Addiction Medicine a. (n.d.). *Public policy statements*. Retrieved October 31, 2021, from https://www.asam.org/advocacy/find-a-policy-statement

American Society of Addiction Medicine b. (n.d.). *Snapshot*. Retrieved October 21, 2021, from https://www.asamcontinuum.org/knowledgebase/what-are-the-asam-levels-of-care/

Alcoff, L. M. (1998). What should white people do? *Hypatia, 13*(3), 6–26. 10.1111/j.1527-2001.1998.tb01367.x

Aldridge, R. W., Story, A., Hwang, S. W., Nordentoft, M., Luchenski, S. A., Hartwell, G., Tweed, E. J., Lewer, D., Vittal Katikireddi, S., & Hayward, A. C. (2018). Morbidity and mortality in homeless individuals, prisoners, sex workers, and individuals with substance use disorders in high-income countries: A systematic review and meta-analysis. *Lancet (London, England), 391*(10117), 241–250. 10.1016/S0140-6736(17)31869-X

American Psychiatric Association. (2013). *Diagnostic and statistical manual of mental disorders (DSM-5®)*. American Psychiatric Publishing. http://ebookcentral.proquest.com/lib/uncg/detail.action?docID=1811753

ASTHO. (2017). *Public health approaches to preventing substance misuse and addictions | State public health | ASTHO*. https://www.astho.org/addictions/

Austin, A. E., Shiue, K. Y., Naumann, R. B., Figgatt, M. C., Gest, C., & Shanahan, M. E. (2021). Associations of housing stress with later substance use outcomes: A systematic review. *Addictive Behaviors, 123*, 107076. 10.1016/j.addbeh.2021.107076

Baranyi, G., Scholl, C., Fazel, S., Patel, V., Priebe, S., & Mundt, A. P. (2019). Severe mental illness and substance use disorders in prisoners in low-income and middle-income countries: A systematic review and meta-analysis of prevalence studies. *The Lancet. Global Health, 7*(4), e461–e471. 10.1016/S2214-109X(18)30539-4

Bolinski, R., Ellis, K., Zahnd, W. E., Walters, S., McLuckie, C., Schneider, J., Rodriguez, C., Ezell, J., Friedman, S. R., Pho, M., & Jenkins, W. D. (2019). Social norms associated with nonmedical opioid use in rural communities: A systematic review. *Translational Behavioral Medicine, 9*(6), 1224–1232. 10.1093/tbm/ibz129

California Health Care Foundation (2018). California Health Care Almanac: Substance Use in California. A look at addiction treatment. https://www.chcf.org/wp-content/uploads/2018/09/SubstanceUseDisorderAlmanac2018.pdf

Castaldelli-Maia, J. M., Marziali, M. E., Lu, Z., & Martins, S. S. (2021). Investigating the effect of national government physical distancing measures on depression and anxiety during the COVID-19 pandemic through meta-analysis and meta-regression. *Psychological Medicine, 51*(6), 881–893. 10.1017/S0033291721000933

Carpenter, C. S., McClellan, C. B., & Rees, I. R. (2017). Economic conditions, illicit drug use, and substance use disorders in the United States. *Journal of Health Economics, 52*, 63–73. 10.1016/j.jhealeco.2016.12.009

Dennis, M., Babor, T. F., Roebuck, M. C., & Donaldson, J. (2002). Changing the focus: The case for recognizing and treating cannabis use disorders. *Addiction (Abingdon, England), 97*(Suppl 1), 4–15. 10.1046/j.1360-0443.97.s01.10.x

Escohotado, A. (1999). *A brief history of drugs: From the stone age to the stoned age*. Park Street Press.

Funk, R. R., McDermeit, M., Godley, S. H., & Adams, L. (2003). Maltreatment issues by level of adolescent substance abuse treatment: The extent of the problem at intake and relationship to early outcomes. *Child Maltreatment, 8*(1), 36–45. 10.1177/1077559502239607

Gilbert, P. A., Pass, L. E., Keuroghlian, A. S., Greenfield, T. K., & Reisner, S. L. (2018). Alcohol research with transgender populations: A systematic review and recommendations to strengthen future studies. *Drug and Alcohol Dependence, 186*, 138–146. 10.1016/j.drugalcdep.2018.01.016

Grant, B. F., Goldstein, R. B., Saha, T. D., Chou, S. P., Jung, J., Zhang, H., Pickering, R. P., Ruan, W. J., Smith, S. M., Huang, B., & Hasin, D. S. (2015). Epidemiology of DSM-5 alcohol use disorder: Results from the national epidemiologic survey on alcohol and related conditions III. *JAMA Psychiatry, 72*(8), 757–766. 10.1001/jamapsychiatry.2015.0584

Hakobyan, S., Vazirian, S., Lee-Cheong, S., Krausz, M., Honer, W. G., & Schutz, C. G. (2020). Concurrent disorder management guidelines. Systematic review. *Journal of Clinical Medicine, 9*(8), 2406. 10.3390/jcm9082406

Henkel, D. (2011). Unemployment and substance use: A review of the literature (1990-2010). *Current Drug Abuse Reviews, 4*(1), 4–27. 10.2174/1874473711104010004

Javed, B., Sarwer, A., Soto, E. B., & Mashwani, Z. (2020). The coronavirus (COVID-19) pandemic's impact on mental health. *The International Journal of Health Planning and Management*, 10.1002/hpm.3008. 10.1002/hpm.3008

Jensen, E., Gerber, J., & Mosher, C. (2004). Social consequences of the war on drugs: The legacy of failed policy. *Criminal Justice Policy Review*, 15, 100–121. 10.1177/08874 03403255315

Kaskutas, L. A., Borkman, T. J., Laudet, A., Ritter, L. A., Witbrodt, J., Subbaraman, M. S., Stunz, A., & Bond, J. (2014). Elements that define recovery: The experiential perspective. *Journal of Studies on Alcohol and Drugs*, 75(6), 999–1010. 10.15288/jsad.2014.75.999

Kelley, A., (2021). *Get back on your bike*. https://www.allysonkelleypllc.com/post/recovery-get-back-on-your-bike

Khoury, L., Tang, Y. L., Bradley, B., Cubells, J. F., & Ressler, K. J. (2010). Substance use, childhood traumatic experience, and posttraumatic stress disorder in an urban civilian population. *Depression and Anxiety*, 27(12), 1077–1086. 10.1002/da.20751

Lewer, D., Meier, P., Beard, E., Boniface, S., & Kaner, E. (2016). Unravelling the alcohol harm paradox: A population-based study of social gradients across very heavy drinking thresholds. *BMC Public Health*, 16, 599. 10.1186/s12889-016-3265-9

Mamun, M. A., Sakib, N., Gozal, D., Bhuiyan, A. I., Hossain, S., Bodrud-Doza, M., Al Mamun, F., Hosen, I., Safiq, M. B., Abdullah, A. H., Sarker, M. A., Rayhan, I., Sikder, M. T., Muhit, M., Lin, C.-Y., Griffiths, M. D., & Pakpour, A. H. (2021). The COVID-19 pandemic and serious psychological consequences in Bangladesh: A population-based nationwide study. *Journal of Affective Disorders*, 279, 462–472. 10.1016/j.jad.2020.10.036

Mann, K. (2000). One hundred years of alcoholism: The twentieth century. *Alcohol and Alcoholism*, 35(1), 10–15. 10.1093/alcalc/35.1.10

Marel, C., Mills, K. L., & Teesson, M. (2021). Substance use, mental disorders and COVID-19: A volatile mix. *Current Opinion in Psychiatry*, 34(4), 351–356. 10.1097/YCO.0000000000000707

Martin, C., Steinley, D., Verges, A., & Sher, K. (2011). Letter to the editor: The proposed 2/11 symptom algorithm for DSM-5 substance-use disorders is too lenient. *Psychological Medicine*, 41(9), 2008–2010. 10.1017/S0033291711000717

McKnight-Eily, L. R., Okoro, C. A., Strine, T. W., Verlenden, J., Hollis, N. D., Njai, R., Mitchell, E. W., Board, A., Puddy, R., & Thomas, C. (2021). Racial and ethnic disparities in the prevalence of stress and worry, mental health conditions, and increased substance use among adults during the COVID-19 Pandemic—United States, April and May 2020. *Morbidity and Mortality Weekly Report*, 70(5), 162–166. 10.15585/mmwr.mm7005a3

McLellan, A. (2017). Substance misuse and substance use disorders: why do they matter in healthcare? *Transactions of the American Clinical and Climatological Association*, 128, 112–130. https://www.ncbi.nlm.nih.gov/pmc/articles/PMC5525418/

National Center for Drug Abuse Statistics. (2021). Drug abuse statistics. https://drugabusestatistics.org/

Nochaiwong, S., Ruengorn, C., Thavorn, K., Hutton, B., Awiphan, R., Phosuya, C., Ruanta, Y., Wongpakaran, N., & Wongpakaran, T. (2021). Global prevalence of mental health issues among the general population during the coronavirus disease-2019 pandemic: A systematic review and meta-analysis. *Scientific Reports*, 11(1), 10173. 10.1038/s41598-021-89700-8

Olson, S., & Gerstein, D. R. (1985). Drinking in America. In *Alcohol in America: Taking Action to Prevent Abuse*. National Academies Press (US). https://www.ncbi.nlm.nih. gov/books/NBK217463/

Polcin, D. L., Korcha, R. A., Bond, J., & Galloway, G. (2010). Sober living houses for alcohol and drug dependence: 18-month outcomes. *Journal of Substance Abuse Treatment, 38*(4), 356–365. 10.1016/j.jsat.2010.02.003

Probst, C., Kilian, C., Sanchez, S., Lange, S., & Rehm, J. (2020). The role of alcohol use and drinking patterns in socioeconomic inequalities in mortality: A systematic review. *The Lancet. Public Health, 5*(6), e324–e332. 10.1016/S2468-2667(20)30052-9

Richmond-Rakerd, L. S., Slutske, W. S., & Wood, P. K. (2017). Age of initiation and substance use progression: A multivariate latent growth analysis. *Psychology of Addictive Behaviors: Journal of the Society of Psychologists in Addictive Behaviors, 31*(6), 664–675. 10.1037/adb0000304

Ritchie, H., & Roser, M. (2018). Mental health. *Our World in Data.* https:// ourworldindata.org/mental-health

Schick, M. R., Spillane, N. S., & Hostetler, K. L. (2020). A call to action: A systematic review examining the failure to include females and members of minoritized racial/ ethnic groups in clinical trials of pharmacological treatments for alcohol use disorder. *Alcoholism: Clinical and Experimental Research, 44*(10), 1933–1951. 10.1111/acer.14440

Schuler, M. S., Rice, C. E., Evans-Polce, R. J., & Collins, R. (2018). Disparities in substance use behaviors and disorders among adult sexual minorities by age, gender, and sexual identity. *Drug and Alcohol Dependence, 189*, 139–146. 10.1016/j. drugalcdep.2018.05.008

Sher, K., Wood, M., Wood, P., & Raskin, G. (1996). Alcohol outcome expectancies and alcohol use: A latent variable cross- lagged panel study. *Journal of Abnormal Psychology, 105*, 561–574. 10.1037//0021-843X.105.4.561

Slade, M., & Wallace, G. (2017). Recovery and mental health. In M. Slade, L. Oades, & A. Jarden (Eds.), *Wellbeing, recovery and mental health* (1st ed., pp. 24–34). Cambridge University Press. 10.1017/9781316339275.004

Stanis, J. J., & Andersen, S. L. (2014). Reducing substance use during adolescence: A translational framework for prevention. *Psychopharmacology, 231*(8), 1437–1453. 10.1007/s00213-013-3393-1

Substance Abuse and Mental Health Services Administration & Healthy People. (n.d.). *Leading health indicators, substance abuse.* Retrieved October 12, 2021, from https://www. healthypeople.gov/2020/leading-health-indicators/2020-lhi-topics/Substance-Abuse

Substance Abuse and Mental Health Services Administration & Office of the Surgeon General. (2017). Vision for the future: A public health approach. In *Facing Addiction in America: The Surgeon General's Report on Alcohol, Drugs, and Health [Internet]*. US Department of Health and Human Services. https://www.ncbi.nlm.nih.gov/books/ NBK424861/

Substance Abuse and Mental Health Services Administration. (2019). *2019 NSDUH annual national report | CBHSQ data.* https://www.samhsa.gov/data/report/2019-nsduh-annual-national-report

Torales, J., O'Higgins, M., Castaldelli-Maia, J. M., & Ventriglio, A. (2020). The out-break of COVID-19 coronavirus and its impact on global mental health. *International Journal of Social Psychiatry, 66*(4), 317–320. 10.1177/0020764020915212

Vaeth, P. A. C., Wang-Schweig, M., & Caetano, R. (2017). Drinking, alcohol use disorder, and treatment access and utilization among U.S. racial/ethnic groups. *Alcoholism, Clinical and Experimental Research, 41*(1), 6–19. 10.1111/acer.13285

van Draanen, J. (2017). Introducing reflexivity to evaluation practice: An in-depth case study. *American Journal of Evaluation, 38*(3), 360–375. 10.1177/1098214016668401

Volkow, N. D. (2020). Collision of the COVID-19 and addiction epidemics. *Annals of Internal Medicine, 173*(1), 61–62. 10.7326/M20-1212

Volkow, N. D., Koob, G. F., & McLellan, A. T. (2016). Neurobiologic advances from the brain disease model of addiction. *The New England Journal of Medicine, 374*(4), 363–371. 10.1056/NEJMra1511480

Volkow, N. D., Poznyak, V., Saxena, S., & Gerra, G. (2017). Drug use disorders: Impact of a public health rather than a criminal justice approach. *World Psychiatry, 16*(2), 213–214. 10.1002/wps.20428

Wang, J., & Geng, L. (2019). Effects of socioeconomic status on physical and psychological health: Lifestyle as a mediator. *International Journal of Environmental Research and Public Health, 16*(2), 281. 10.3390/ijerph16020281

World Health Organization. (2018). *Global status report on alcohol and health 2018.* World Health Organization. https://apps.who.int/iris/handle/10665/274603

World Health Organization. (2019). *Suicide rates.* https://www.who.int/data/maternal-newborn-child-adolescent-ageing/advisory-groups/gama/gama-advisory-group-members

Zapolski, T. C. B., Pedersen, S. L., McCarthy, D. M., & Smith, G. T. (2014). Less drinking, yet more problems: Understanding African American drinking and related problems. *Psychological Bulletin, 140*(1), 188–223. 10.1037/a0032113

2 The Research and Theories on Mental Health and Substance Abuse Treatment

CONTENTS

DOI: 10.4324/9781003290728-2

Learning Objectives

After reading this chapter you should be able to ...

1. List research and theories used in treatment settings
2. Differentiate frameworks, theories, and models and their use in evaluation and research
3. Discuss theories that support a social justice frame and health equity lens in treatment contexts

As a researcher, storyteller, and person with the lived experience of recovery, I see the importance of research and theories on mental health and substance use. Without research or theory, we would not know what works, what does not, for whom, and when. The public health approach that we learned about in Chapter 1 is evident in the research and theories about mental health and substance abuse treatment presented and every step (surveillance, understanding, evaluation, and effectiveness) is demonstrated in the collective efforts of researchers, policy makers, evaluators, and clinicians.

Many Paths to Recovery and Evaluation

It is essential to recognize that there are many paths to recovery, and many paths to evaluating treatment programs. Various kinds of evidence generated by researchers and evaluators tell us what works and what does not. However, most of the research and theories on treatment are based on western biomedical models and approaches, and a post-positivist perspective about what constitutes evidence, effectiveness, and validity. One of my favorite quotes by Albert Einstein is that not everything that can be counted counts, and not everything that counts can be counted. Although this discussion is beyond the scope of this text, it is important to consider that most of what we know about recovery comes from researchers and clinicians working within a clinical setting and conceptualized based on their theories. There is an entire pandoras box of approaches that take place outside the research and clinical realm that are effective. With this framing in mind, in this chapter we are going to explore what we know about research and theories, both are essential because they inform evidence, support policy, and overall improve treatment effectiveness.

A socioecological model (SEM) includes public policy/society, community, organizational, interpersonal, and individual/self (patients). Within these levels there are structures, practices, and norms that influence how treatment programs are implemented, and therefore how research, theories, and evaluation happens. Here are some examples of research and evaluation topics organized within the SEM.

- **Public policy, social and cultural norms**
  Evaluators may explore the cost of services, access to services, funding, policies, protocols, practices, laws, criminalization of MHSUD, or equity.
  Evaluators may explore patient centered care, the use of evidence-based practices, media influences and reach, government involvement, or regulations.
- **Community**
  Evaluators may explore neighborhoods, schools, workplaces, social contexts, religious organizations, stigma, social norms, community organization, positions of leaders, cultural norms.
- **Organizational/Institutional/Systems**
  Evaluators may explore healthcare and structures of MHSUD system, practices within the system. Patient treatment, patient communication, stereotypes, discrimination.
  Evaluators may work in partnership with faith-based organizations, recovery organizations, non-profit organizations, county, state, federal programs, or private organizations
- **Interpersonal/Network**
  Evaluators may explore relationships and power equity, social support and trust, relationship satisfaction, communication levels, social networks, coalitions, and capital.
- **Individual**
  Evaluators may collect information about individuals such as age, education, income, attitudes, beliefs, trauma, values, mental health history. In addition, evaluators may document knowledge, risk perception, emotions, denial status, readiness to change, physical health, self-efficacy, perceived social norms, control, beliefs, outcome expectancies, and empowerment constructs.

One public health model to explore the plethora of research and theories on treatment approaches is Bronfenbrenner's work on the **ecology of human development** (1979). His work outlines the overlap of processes and systems and how they impact individuals, families, communities, institutions, and nations (Bronfenbrenner, 1979). Researchers have applied the ecological perspective to research and treatment programs to explore addiction and the interactions that occur at each level. **Chronosystem.** Historical context and changes in environments over time. Wars, disasters, pandemics, recessions. **Macrosystem.** Cultural, political, economic, and social contexts. Technology, treatment funding, information uptake. **Exosystem.** Interactions between at least two environments. Legislative decisions influence policy. **Mesosystem.**

Interactions between two or more environments where individuals exist. Home, school, work, neighborhood, church, medical care. **Microsystem.** In-person interactions between individual and environment. Family, friends, peers, neighbors. **Individual** person,client,and their lived experiences.

The majority of MHSUD prevention efforts have focused on individuals and changes in attitudes, knowledge, and beliefs. Public health calls for a broader, multi-pronged approach, where the focus is on changing conditions at all levels that increase behaviors that place individuals at risk for MHSUD. Previous research indicates that policy change, evidence-based practices, and changing social norms can reduce the prevalence and incidence of SUD (Ballard et al., 2021). We will review policies, systems, and environments (PSE) related to SUD in Chapter 6.

Public Health Takeaway- Prevention and intervention approaches must focus on improving conditions, environments, and social capital **rather than sobriety or abstinence**. History, culture, politics, home, school, work, healthcare, friends, and peers can support holistic and ecological treatment approach.

With the SEM and PSE frameworks in mind, it is essential to consider how research informs evidence-based practices (EBPs). Let's begin by reviewing what EBPs are and how researchers develop EBPs to inform practice about what constitutes effectiveness.

Evidence-Based Practices (EBP)

EBPs have been used for more than 25 years with researchers, policy makers, and programs promoting their use with the overall goal of improving treatment outcomes for mental health and substance abuse. Developers of the movement created the following criteria for EBPs: 1) a minimum of two controlled group design or a large series of single case design studies, 2) a minimum of two investigators, 3) clinicians with uniform training and adherence, and 4) long term outcome measures beyond the end of treatment intervention. Researchers and policy advocates criticized the EBP movement because it failed to address the unique characteristics of the intervention population, for example the age, context, and community. To address these criticisms, Substance Abuse and Mental Health Services Administration (SAMSHA) developed practice-based evidence (PBE). SAMHSA's goal was to expand definitions and go beyond empirical evidence. SAMSHA advocated for evidence that is defined by the persons involved in the intervention, including clinicians, youth, families, and program staff (Kelley et al., 2017).

SAMHSA also developed a strategic initiative for advancing behavioral health to prevent substance abuse and mental illness with a focus on high risk populations (GAO, n.d.). SAMSHA along with researchers, clinicians, and treatment programs embrace EBPs and PBEs as a primary method for addressing substance abuse and advancing behavioral health.

Practice-Based Evidence (PBE)

PBE's are different that EBPs because they are culturally relevant and responsive to the needs of specific communities—this often means that what works for one program may not work for another. However, PBE's have been criticized because there are no clear definitions or parameters on what constitutes a PBE and when it is appropriate for use, and for whom. Proponents have responded by defining PBEs as, "a useful and effective category of interventions, characteristic, and conditions that emerge either alone or in combination that may delineate types of PBE practices categorized as community valued, culturally and socially embedded, heretofore unaddressed community/population conditions, and emergency issues." (Hoagwood & Johnson, 2003). SAMSHA reports that PBEs were developed to both support and criticize EBPs because they open up a "black box" of an intervention and describe formative assessment components such as the day to day operations of a program, data collection, participants, and qualitative data that are meaningful in determining outcomes associated with constructs of interest (SAMSHA, ND).

Best Practices

SAMHSA developed a registry or EBPs in 1977 named the National Registry of Evidence-based Programs and Practices (NREPP). This registry outlined empirically driven interventions for behavioral health issues to treat MI and SUD. Developers and users of NREPP were shocked in 2018 when the White House decided they would no longer fund the project (SAMHSA & the Peter G Dodge Foundation, n.d.). SAMHSA now maintains a best-practices website with reports and guides on effective prevention and intervention approaches.

Evidence

Before we begin this section I want to bring your attention to the concept of **non-quantifiable evidence**. This type of evidence involves the spiritual realm, things that we experience, feel, or believe, that cannot be articulated with numbers or sometimes words. One of the reasons why I want you to think about this concept early in the text, is that many people recover without treatment. Some describe this as a natural recovery, a spiritual transformation, an awakening, that is not quantified (or at least not well). Early in my career I was fascinated with the concepts of the butterfly effect and chaos theory. Both gave me solace when something could not be rationally or realistically explained. Influenced by chaos theory, the **butterfly effect** occurs with the flap of a butterfly's wings. The flapping of wings, at one point in space and time, could cause a tornado somewhere else. Researchers have used the butterfly effect as a metaphor, and to describe self-care and compassion for others (Wilkund Gustin & Wagner, 2013). With this understanding, let's consider quantifiable evidence.

Scientific evidence is generated by researchers (and others). There are different approaches for synthesizing evidence in clinical settings, and in public health practice. The Centers for Disease Control and Prevention and Frieden and colleagues led the Evidence Project which calls for evidence-based decision making based on the best available **research evidence, contextual evidence, and experiential evidence** (Frieden et al., 2011.). **Research evidence** is information from scientific inquiry used to determine if a program, policy, or intervention achieved intended outcomes. Contextual evidence includes measurable factors in a community that may impact outcomes like history, organizational capacity, and social norms. **Experiential evidence** is the collective knowledge and perspectives of individuals and experts (Frieden et al., 2011).

Public Health Takeaway- Recognize that researchers, policy makers, evaluators, and clinicians have different ideas about evidence. Consider multiple forms of evidence (even non-quantifiable evidence) involved in evidence-based decision making. Consider the rigor and standards of available research, ways to identify and collect evidence, and stages of evidence-based decision making (step 3).

The US Surgeon General's Report on Alcohol, Drugs, and Health (2018) synthesized evidence using Frieden's approach. The Surgeon General's Report outlines four MHSUD areas, the evidence base for each, and recommendations for public health.

Early Intervention, Treatment, and Management of SUD

- Evidence suggests that medications are effective in treating SUD, but medications are widely underutilized. Evidence also suggests that brief interventions and screening work for individuals with mild AUD and possibly drug use disorders. Treatment for SUD is cost effective.
- Treatment and management of SUD should be similar as those for other chronic illnesses, improving overall health and functional status.
- Behavioral therapies can be effective when using evidence-based approaches (EBs), but researchers report issues with fidelity and limited use.
- Promising evidence demonstrates that electronic technologies like electronic health records and telehealth may improve access, engagement, retention, and support for individuals with SUD (US Surgeon General, 2018).

The Neurobiology of Substance Use, Misuse, and Addiction

- Evidence suggests that addiction to alcohol and drugs is a brain disease.
- Addiction occurs in a three-stage cycle (binge/intoxication, withdrawal/ negative affect, and preoccupation/anticipation). Evidence suggests that this cycle modifies brain functioning which limits an individual's ability to control use.
- Addiction impacts three areas of the brain: the basal ganglia, extended amygdala, and prefrontal cortex. Impacts result in substance associated cues

to find substances, reduced sensitivity of brain systems, and reduced functioning of brain executive control systems (that regulate decision making, actions, emotions, and impulses).

- Impacts to the brain are observable, even when an individual stops using substances.
- Adolescence is a critical at risk period for substance use and addiction, the adolescent brain is not fully developed placing them at greater risk (US Surgeon General, 2018).

Prevention Programs and Policies

- Evidence outlines the risk and protective factors associated with substance use and misuse. These factors are similar based on gender, race and ethnicity, and income.
- Prevention programs are cost-effective and may be implemented at any time throughout the lifespan.
- Communities may experience different risk and protective factors; prevention and policy efforts must elevate these needs and address them with EBIs.
- Policies that reduce alcohol availability and increase the costs of alcohol are effective.
- Laws targeting driving under the influence are effective in reducing alcohol-related crash fatalities (US Surgeon General, 2018).

Recovery and Wellness

- Evidence suggests that almost 50% of adults with a previous SUD are in stable remission (more than 1 year).
- Mutual aid groups and recovery support organizations and programs are instrumental in promoting recovery from SUD in the U.S.
- Evidence suggests that 12-step mutual aid groups focused on alcohol and 12-step facilitated interventions are effective.
- There is promising evidence for recovery supports, and a key issue is the lack of evidence or studies on recovery support services (US Surgeon General, 2018).

Public Health Takeaway- The US Surgeon General outlines a growing body of evidence related to early intervention, prevention, policies, recovery and wellness. Public health initiatives must consider all forms of evidence while advocating for equity in evidence-based treatments for all.

With this evidence in mind, let's consider how evidence, therapies, and approaches are used with MHSUD populations. Evidence-based approaches for drug treatment can include behavioral therapy (such as cognitive-behavioral therapy or contingency management), medications, or a combination of behavioral and medical treatments. Notably, many of the EBs for SUD can also be used for MH or individuals with co-occurring disorders (Pacheco et al., 2013).

NIDA identified principles of drug abuse treatment that may be useful in the evaluation of MHSU programs and treatment efforts (2018).

- Addiction is a complex but treatable disease that affects brain function and behavior.
- No single treatment is appropriate for everyone.
- Treatment needs to be readily available.
- Effective treatment attends to multiple needs of the individual, not just his or her drug abuse. Remaining in treatment for an adequate period of time is critical.
- Behavioral therapies—including individual, family, or group counseling—are the most commonly used forms of drug abuse treatment.
- Medications are an essential element of treatment for many patients, especially when combined with counseling and other behavioral therapies.
- An individual's treatment and services plan must be assessed continually and modified as necessary to ensure that it meets his or her changing needs.
- Many drug-addicted individuals also have other mental disorders.
- Medically assisted detoxification is only the first stage of addiction treatment and by itself does little to change long-term drug abuse.
- Treatment does not need to be voluntary to be effective.
- Drug use during treatment must be monitored continuously, as lapses during treatment do occur.

Below is a list of some evidence-based treatment modalities for MHSUD or co-occurring disorders from the published literature. This list is not comprehensive, and it does not include all evidence-based treatments.

Acceptance and Commitment Therapy is an EB therapy model that includes, strategies of detaching from inner experiences by relating to them differently; learning how to accept thoughts and feelings without trying to change their form or frequency; mindfulness to stay in the present moment; self-understanding to let go of concrete and inflexible thoughts or ideas about oneself; learning what is important to oneself in regard to values; and committed action and empowerment for behavioral change (Bluett et al., 2014; Worley, 2020).

Cognitive-behavioral therapy (CBT) focuses on how thoughts affect behavior and these behaviors impact emotions (Beck Institute, n.d.; Thoma et al., 2015). EB CBT practices to address SUMH include strategies such as learning how to delay and distract cravings by engaging in constructive activities, journaling, communicating with others, going to meetings, and other positive strategies by which to ride out the wave of craving until it subsides. A hallmark of CBT is to address any negative thinking patterns and considering positive thinking and responses through journaling. CBT strategies also include considering the consequences of substance use and identifying elevated risk situations. CBT may involve role-playing and being in situations where an individual learns how to navigate cravings, peer pressure, and stressful environments. CBT stresses the importance of healthy supportive interactions like peer support groups and talking circles along with physical, mental, emotional, and spiritual wellbeing (Worley, 2020). Generally, treatment and follow-up times range between 0 and 9 months. There is strong evidence that CBT is effective and outcomes associated with CBT include decreases in substance use, reductions in severity of PTSD and depressive symptoms, and reductions in trauma associated cognitions (Curry et al., 2003; Fortuna et al., 2018).

Dialectical Behavioral Therapy (DBT) is an EB strategy that builds skills in patients to reduce or stop use. DBT combines mindfulness, distress tolerance, self-regulation, and interpersonal development. One category of DBT is contingency management (CM) (Walter & Petry, 2016). CM identifies people, places, objects, or activities that reinforce abstinence (Worley, 2020).

Eye movement desensitization reprocessing (EMDR) is based on an adaptive information processing (AIP) model that addresses dysfunctional stored and unprocessed memories that may be the cause of a number of mental disorders, including posttraumatic stress disorder (PTSD), mood disorders, chronic pain, eating disorders, addiction, and various others (Wilson et al., 2018).

Mindfulness-based interventions (MBI) are EB approaches that encourage individuals to experience the present moment without judgement, stress, or thinking. Research on MBI shows that it supports self-regulation, decreasing the size and activity of the amygdala which relates to worry and anxiety. Overall MBI reduces emotional reactivity and research indicates it reduces cravings for substance use (Fortuna et al., 2018; Grant et al., 2017).

Multidimensional Family Therapy (MDFT) is a manualized, family-focused approach to treat youth with substance misuse, SUD, and co-occurring mental and behavioral health problems. Outcomes associated with MDFT include reductions in problems associated with SU, reductions in past 30-day SU, and reductions in internalization of MH symptoms (Liddle et al., 2018).

Pharmacotherapy involves medications approved by the Federal Drug Administration to treat MHSU needs. Pharmacotherapy treatment depends on an individual's age and diagnosis. Often pharmacotherapy treatment is combined with psychotherapy treatment. Although beyond the scope of this text, there are specific pharmacotherapy treatments that evaluators should be aware of. For example, there are three medications approved by the FDA to approve opioid use disorder (OUD). These include buprenorphine, methadone, and naltrexone. Another example is a diagnosis of depression may include the FDA-approved medication of Fluoxetine, also known as Prozac.

Evidence-Based Practices for Co-Occurring Disorders

Research by Flynn and colleagues makes the case for DBT EBs for patients with dual diagnosis (Flynn et al., 2019). Flynn's study reported that DBT resulted in reductions in binge drinking drug use and increases in the use of mindfulness practices and DBT skills. Qualitative data from this study reinforce study outcomes, that DBT is effective and builds skills that address MHSU problems. Another study by Kothgassner and colleagues reports on the efficacy of DBT for adolescent self-harm and suicidal ideation using a systematic review and meta-analysis process (Kothgassner et al., 2021). In this review, DBT decreased adolescent self-harm and suicidal ideation, but did not reduce symptoms of borderline personality disorder (BPD).

Cochrane Review

One of the greatest resources available, informed by research and evaluation is the Cochrane Review database (www.cochrane.org). Cochrane produces rigorous reviews of research in human health care and policy and shares it with the world. I went to the Cochrane website, typed in drug addiction to search the evidence and 52 results appeared (in .049 seconds which is fast). As an evaluator and researcher of treatment programs I can look at these reviews and see what evidence is available to support a selected treatment approach and use this to frame the evaluation. For example, I am interested in approaches used to evaluate psychosocial interventions like talking therapies and the evidence available to support their use. Here are some examples from the Cochrane review.

Review of Psychosocial Interventions for Drug Use and Alcohol Problems

Klimas and colleagues wanted to know which talking therapies work for people who use drugs and also have alcohol problems. They found seven studies that explored five different talking therapies among 825 people with drug problems. Talking therapies included Cognitive-behavioral coping skills training, twelve-step programs, motivational interviewing (MI), brief motivational interviewing (BMI) and brief interventions based on MI but shorter (2018). Their results completely disappointed me, talking therapies led to no difference or small differences in outcomes assessed like abstinence, reduced drinking, and substance use (Klimas et al., 2018). Bummer. As an evaluator and researcher, it is essential to consider the treatment approach, the evidence available, outcomes assessed, and population.

Review of School-Based Prevention for Illicit Drug Use

School-based efforts to prevent illicit drug use are widely used throughout the United States and globe, yet I have always wondered if they are actually effective. We all know the DARE program was not effective, but that is another story (Kelley, 2020). Cochrane published their review of school-based prevention for illicit drug use and found 51 studies with 127,146 participants enrolled. The majority of studies compared adopting a social competence approach to a usual curricula approach. Other studies compared social influence approaches with usual curricula. Most studies were implemented with sixth or seventh grade students in the US. Interventions were interactive and varied in duration. Follow-up ranged from immediately following the intervention to 10 years after the intervention. Programs based on social influence showed weak effects that were not significant. Programs that combined social competence and social influence approaches fared better with preventing marijuana use longer and preventing drug use. Knowledge-based interventions showed no differences, other than knowledge but knowledge does not prevent illicit drug use. Researchers recommended school-based prevention efforts combined with more comprehensive prevention approaches due to the small effects noted in these studies (Faggiano et al., 2014).

Review of Alcoholics Anonymous (AA) and Other 12-Step Programs for AUD

AUD is a significant public health problem. AA and 12-step programs/mutual aid groups help individuals recover. Cochrane published a review of these programs and found 27 studies with 10,565 participants enrolled. Studies varied in their design, where some explored treatment delivery, others compared AA with other treatments like Cognitive Behavioral Therapy (CBT). Most studies were funded by the National Institutes of Health, the Department of Veterans Affairs, and other organizations. Reviewers found that overall AA interventions produced higher rates over longer periods of time of continuous abstinence. They found that AA may be preferred over other treatments (e.g., CBT). AA reduces the intensity of drinking and results in significant cost savings. Researchers call for clinically-delivered 12-step programs to increase participation in AA groups. Notably, AA groups continue beyond the clinical treatment intervention time period, resulting in longer-term support for individuals with AUD (Kelly et al., 2020).

Review of Psychosocial Interventions for Cannabis/Marijuana Use Disorder

Cannabis use disorder is pervasive in the United States impacting three out of every 10 individuals who use marijuana (Hasin et al., 2015). Cochrane published a review of 23 studies including 4,045 participants with frequent cannabis use. The average age of participants was 28.2 years, and most were male. Studies were conducted in the United States, Germany, Australia, Brazil, Canada, Switzerland, and Ireland. Published studies reviewed several psychosocial intervention types including cognitive-behavioral therapy (CBT), motivational enhancement therapy (MET), a combination of MET and CBT (MET + CBT), contingency management (CM), social support, mindfulness, and drug education and counseling. Reviewers found that psychosocial interventions in community and outpatient settings are difficult to implement. However, CBT individual and group sessions and MET in individual sessions were most commonly used in this population. Both CBT and MET demonstrated effectiveness. Psychosocial treatment consistently demonstrated effectiveness in studies compared with individuals who did not receive treatment. Comparison studies reviewed by Cochrane found that participants receiving any intervention reported lessdays of cannabis use and fewer dependence symptoms than individuals who did not receive interventions. Three of the studies Cochrane reviewed found that there were no differences in the psychosocial intervention group compared with the control group. Results for CM interventions were mixed, with slight improvements in use frequency and severity of dependences. Researchers felt that these CM interventions were combined with other CBT or MET+CBT which makes it difficult to isolate the effects of CM on desired outcomes. Reviewers advocate for better quality evidence and call for consistent assessment measures. Drop-out rates and loss to follow-up threaten the overall evidence for psychosocial interventions that address cannabis use disorder (Gates, et al., 2016).

Public Health Takeaway- The Cochrane Review makes it easy to find systematic studies of treatment approaches. Evaluators and public health advocates must be careful when relying only on Cochrane's evidence which is grounded in a post-positivist view about what constitutes evidence or truth.

Theories

I remember someone told me once that policies are just theories about what we think will happen. That has always stuck with me as I move between theory, policy, evidence, and practice as an evaluator, researcher, storyteller, and writer.

"The hallmark of a scientific model is that it provides a framework within which the scientific method may be applied. The value of a scientific model is measured not by whether it is right or wrong but how useful it is. It is modified or discarded when it no longer helps generate and test new knowledge." - Engel, 1980 p. 543.

Theories and Models about Addiction

The famous (and controversial) **Rat Park** experiments in the 1970s by Bruce K Alexander showed us the power of community, connection, and conditions (Gage & Sumnall, 2019). Alexander reported that rats living in a social environment (park) were less likely to use morphine than rats living in an isolated environment (without the park). Researchers replicated variations of the rat park experiment to test theories and assumptions about addiction. One study explored housing (rat park) and gender differences and morphine consumption. Results from the 1978 study found that isolated rats drank more than social rats and females drank more morphine than males (Alexander et al., 1978). The second study explored housing (via rat parks) and gender effects on preference for morphine-sucrose (sugar) solutions in rats (1972). Findings from this study suggest limited evidence that housing and gender affected high morphine, and low sucrose conditions. A final study in 1981 explored the effect of early and later colony housing on oral injection of morphine in rats (Alexander et al., 1981). Rats living in the rat park consumed less morphine than those living in isolation, even after considering their early life experiences. There was no evidence to suggest that early environments related to increased morphine consumption. A limitation of all rat park experiments is that differences in morphine consumption only occurred under specific conditions and with rats already addicted to morphine, and at specific times in the research process (B. K. Alexander et al., 1978, 1981; Gage & Sumnall, 2019). People are not rats, and the rat park model may not be a true representation of the socioecological factors that contribute to addiction or health and wellbeing. But this research is worth considering when developing public health prevention, intervention, and recovery approaches to MHSUD and conceptualizing recovery communities and how to build health, home, community, and purpose. Another model that we will use in this text is the **disease model of addiction**. It is a casual model showing that when an organ (like the brain) experiences a defect (which is caused by something like drug or alcohol consumption), and symptoms of the disease occur (addiction). Based on the concept that there are genetic and biological factors that contribute to addiction as a brain disease, proponents of the disease model call for cures through abstinence, 12-step models, and medical treatment. A key factor in calling addiction a disease rather than something else (moral problem, family problem, personality problem, choice), is that by calling it a disease individuals can be treated within a healthcare system, and in most cases healthcare systems can be reimbursed for the treatment they provide. However, critics of the disease model of addiction feel that it overly pathologizes the brain and the person (Pickard, 2017; Lewis, 2015). Moreover, by calling addiction a disease, individuals with addiction may feel helpless, disempowered, and dependent on medical providers and clinicians to cure their disease (Pickard, 2017). Notably, most individuals with addiction do not view themselves as diseased. Mark Lewis promotes a new way of thinking about rat parks, moral and disease models- the **learning model of addiction** (2015). Within this model, Lewis espouses that addiction is the product of learning and development which can be overcome through further learning and development, agency empowerment, self-understanding and environments that create conditions where these characteristics are developed (Lewis, 2015). The **socioecological model** (see Chapter 2) is also useful when exploring public health issues that have a behavioral health component. For example, the causal relationship between drinking and driving under the influence is clear, but drinking is not the only reason why an individual is pulled over for a DUI. Consider the role of relationships (peer influences), the environment and community, and society (norms related to DUI policies and laws and blood alcohol levels).

What is a theory? A **theory** describes what we think will happen based on existing scientific evidence, research, or knowledge (Engel, 1980). Theories can be built or tested and inform practice, hence their importance (McNab & Partridge, 2014). Notably, theories may be based in principles, incorporate laws or concepts, or be used to test a hypothesis. Theories may be implicit or explicit. Use of theory in clinical practice and evaluation helps build an evidence base of causal mechanisms that lead to desired results. Theoretically driven treatment approaches may be tailored based on the target population and setting (Moore & Evans, 2017).

Here are some ways evaluators and clinicians use theories in the evaluation of treatment programs:

Theories to diagnose- clinicians
Theories to explain behaviors - clinicians and evaluators
Theories to test assumptions- evaluators
Theories to guide evaluation (desired outcomes, and theory of change)- evaluators (Trauer, 2010)

Often times the terms theory, model, or framework are used interchangeably, and at times this can be confusing. Table 2.1 outlines characteristics of theories, and models with simplified definitions, uses, and examples.

Using Theory in Evaluation

As evaluators it is essential to understand the use of theory. Clinicians may use theories to guide their diagnosis and develop a treatment plan for an individual. One example is John Bowlby's **Attachment Theory** where attachment is described as a lasting psychological connectedness between human beings. Bowlby posited that attachment was related to separation anxiety and distress in children when they were separated from their caregivers. Attachment theory explains child diagnoses of oppositional defiant disorder, conduct disorder, PTSD, abuse, and neglect.

Table 2.1 Theories, Models, and Frameworks

	Theory	*Model*	*Framework*
Simple definition	Analytical principles or statements	Simplified explanation of a theory	Structure, system, or plan with relationships
Strengths	Provide evidence	Easier to understand	Captures multiple contextual factors
Limitations	Explains, describes but does not provide evidence	Narrow focus	Does not provide explanations
Example	Theory of Planned Behavior (Michie et al., 2011)	Biopsychosocial model (Engel, 1980)	RE-AIM evaluation framework (Glasgow et al., 1999)

Behavior theories such as **Social Cognition Theory and Theory of Reason Action** are common in MHSUD treatment milieu. One of the shortcomings of these theories is that they focus solely on psychological processes and ignore contextual and socioecological factors (community, nation, systems, and structures) that influence one's behavior. While the SEM model presented earlier in this chapter allows us to conceptualizes how these theories might play out on a broader scale, more work is necessary to explore and understand the use and testing of these theories in intervention and program research, and evaluation.

"Addiction is increasingly being described by US researchers and the National Institute on Drug Abuse (NIDA) as a chronic and relapsing brain disease."
- Bell et al., 2014 p. 19

Other commonly used theories in treatment settings include **Stages of Change** (Prochaska & DiClemente, 1983) (Figure 2.1), Theory of Planned Behavior (Ajzen, 1991), and the **medical disease model** which identifies addiction as a medical disorder (Bell et al., 2014). Other models that are not therapeutic but that relate to treatment include moral models such as **Alcoholics Anonymous** (AA) where belief in a higher power is necessary to overcome the disease. Temperance models traced back to the 1840s maintain that an individual is powerless against addiction, abstinence is the only path (See, 2013).

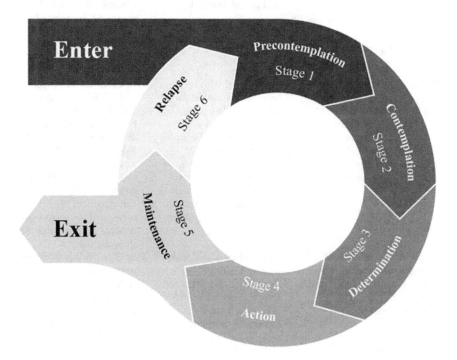

Figure 2.1 Stages of Change Model and Treatment Programs.
(Prochaska & DiClemente, 1983).

As evaluators our focus should be on theories that guide the evaluation process. As an evaluator you might be familiar with the term **Theory of Change (ToC)** and sometimes we refer to ToC as a framework or a model. Existing evidence suggests that before developing a ToC evaluators need to understand what the problem is, how the problem was created, and how the problem persists in certain contexts (Moore & Evans, 2017). Once this understanding is gained, the ToC process involves outlining mental models, considering change theories, exploring existing research and evaluation in similar contexts, and exploring the strengths and weaknesses of the ToC developed and articulated in a model, Table 2.2.

Table 2.2 Theory of Change and Six Stages of Change in Recovery

Stage	Example	Treatment Needs
Pre-contemplation. The individual is not considering change, is aware of few negative consequences, and is unlikely to take action soon.	A functional yet alcohol-dependent individual who drinks himself into a stupor every night but who goes to work every day, performs his job, has no substance abuse-related legal problems, has no health problems, and is still married.	This client needs information linking his problems and potential problems with his substance abuse. A brief intervention might be to educate him about the negative consequences of substance abuse. For example, if he is depressed, he might be told how his alcohol abuse may cause or exacerbate the depression.
Contemplation. The individual is aware of some pros and cons of substance abuse but feels ambivalent about change. This individual has not yet decided to commit to change.	An individual who has received a citation for driving while intoxicated and vows that next time she will not drive when drinking. She is aware of the consequences but makes no commitment to stop drinking, just to not drive after drinking.	This client should explore feelings of ambivalence and the conflicts between her substance abuse and personal values. The brief intervention might seek to increase the client's awareness of the consequences of continued abuse and the benefits of decreasing or stopping use.
Preparation. This stage begins once the individual has decided to change and begins to plan steps toward recovery.	An individual who decides to stop abusing substances and plans to attend counseling, AA, NA, or a formal treatment program.	This client needs work on strengthening commitment. A brief intervention might give the client a list of options for treatment (e.g., inpatient treatment, outpatient

(*Continued*)

Table 2.2 (Continued)

Stage	Example	Treatment Needs
		treatment, 12-Step meetings) from which to choose, then help the client plan how to go about seeking the treatment that is best for him.
Action. The individual tries new behaviors, but these are not yet stable. This stage involves the first active steps toward change.	An individual who goes to counseling and attends meetings but often thinks of using again or may even relapse at times.	This client requires help executing an action plan and may have to work on skills to maintain sobriety. The clinician should acknowledge the client's feelings and experiences as a normal part of recovery. Brief interventions could be applied throughout this stage to prevent relapse.
Maintenance. The individual establishes new behaviors on a long-term basis.	An individual who attends counseling regularly, is actively involved in AA or NA, has a sponsor, may be taking disulfiram (Antabuse), has made new sober friends, and has found new substance-free recreational activities.	This client needs help with relapse prevention. A brief intervention could reassure, evaluate present actions, and redefine long-term sobriety maintenance plans.
Relapse. The individual relapses.	An individual relapses and begins abusing substances and is not attending counseling, AA, NA, or a formal treatment	This client needs help and a brief intervention, and support for long-term sobriety maintenance. plans

Adapted from Prochaska and DiClemente, 1983; Substance Abuse and Mental Health Services Administration, 1999.

There is much more to the ToC process that we can apply to individual and program change, check out Chapter 3 for more information about ToC and logic models. If you are dying to know more about ToC, check out one of my favorite online evaluation resources, Better Evaluation located in the resources section at the end of this chapter.

Systems theory offers a partial solution to the narrow focus of psychological and behavior-focused theories (like a readiness for change model outlined previously), but systems theories are messy and therefore many evaluators and clinicians shy away from their use (Moore & Evans, 2017). The **Biopsychosocial model** (BPS) is one of the most commonly used general systems theories in treatment settings. This model explores biological, social, and psychological factors as they related to MHSUD. **Biological factors** include genetics, disease, injury, hormones, diet, exercise, drugs, alcohol, toxins, and stressors. Social factors may include upbringing, family, peer relationships, poverty, school, media, culture, work, stress, trauma, discrimination, and racism. **Psychological factors** include beliefs, emotions, resilience, coping, emotional intelligence, cognitive biases, behavior, and IQ. The interplay of these factors at various times, settings, context, and stages of life contribute to one's overall mental health and use of substances (for example, substances used in moderation, substance misuse, substance abuse).

General Systems Theory Evaluation Example

Here is an example of a GST approach to the evaluation of a treatment program, Figure 2.2.

The diagram below demonstrates the application of a GST in mental health treatment where boxes represent populations served and contextual factors within the systems are noted by informational context, schools, treatment, evaluation, and the flow of clients into and out of the system.

Hellenic Center for Mental Health and Research (HCMHR) is a public organization in Greece offering a network of mental healthcare services and resources (Katrakazas et al., 2020).

Creators of the HCMHR GST example point to several limitations. The model fails to address legislative, policy, or financial frameworks? HCMHR did not include other evidence-based approaches and treatment programs. HCMHR did not account for patients that are referred to HCMHR but never treated and follow-up procedures. While every model, theory, and approach has limitations, HCMHR is an example of a multi-level, systems theory and approach that may be used to address some of the limitations of narrowly focused behavioral theories.

Social capital theory (SCT) is the actual or perceived potential aggregate resources that are linked to networks of relationships and support (Jason et al., 2020). Researchers utilize SCT to explain and advocate for recovery-support services like peer mentoring, sober living houses, and sober activities. Research supported by SCT indicates that when individuals belong to a social network of abstainers (those who are not using drugs or alcohol) this was one of the strongest predictors of quality of life after treatment (Best et al., 2011; Jason

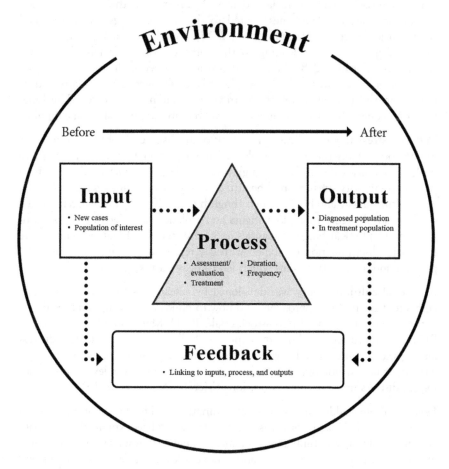

Figure 2.2 General Systems Theory Template Example.

et al., 2020). Theorists believe that these relationships provide social capital that supports an individual's decision to abstain from use.

This section below highlights specific theories used in MHSUD evaluation contexts that address experiences such as stigma, minority stress, discrimination, structural factors, and more.

Critical race theory (CRT) is about relationships between race, racism, and power informed by feminist theory, civil rights, and ethnic studies (Fornili, 2018). Scholars assert that racism happens all of the time and it is normalized, invisible, and ignored in our world (Delgado et al., 2017). Delgado and Stefanic apply CRT to the current war on drugs, with clear evidence of racism in the school to prison pipeline, racialized mass incarceration, the for-profit prison system, and negative outcomes related to the war on drugs on families and communities of color (Delgado et al., 2017). People of color are arrested at higher rates than whites leading to the current crisis of racialized mass incarceration (Fornili, 2018). More than two million people in the US live in a prison or jail and two thirds are people of color (Mauer, 2016). Current drug policies in the United States are destroying communities of color. The long-term consequences of these policies on children and families are immeasurable.

Minority stress theory indicates that stress occurs as a result of being a minority in the form of discrimination, violence, and rejection that leads to negative health outcomes (Meyer, 2003). English and colleagues reviewed the effects of stigma on minority stress, mental health, and substance use among Black, Latino, and multiracial gay and bisexual men (English et al., 2018). This research applied minority stress theory to explore stigma and violence as underlying factors contributing to physical health inequities and substance use. Findings demonstrate that racial discrimination combined with gay rejection sensitivity increased depression and anxiety symptoms which led to heavy drinking.

Relational-cultural theory was developed by researchers to support culturally competent counseling approaches and how to build relationships and resilience within the clinical setting (Comstock et al., 2011). Mereish and Poteat applied RCT to explore relationships, resilience, and alleviating psychological distress among sexual minorities. They found that fostering relationships among people with internalized homophobia may be associated with lower levels of psychological distress under specific conditions (Mereish & Poteat, 2015).

Feminist theory addresses issues of discrimination and exclusion on the basis of sex and gender. In addition, this theory can be used to explore the objectification of women, structural and economic inequality that may result from being a woman, power and oppression, and gender roles and stereotypes. Evans and colleagues developed BREATHE, a black women's feminist therapy treatment approach that supports mental health. BREATHE is unique because it recognizes the unique role and position of Black women in a modern society and how these roles may negatively impact and overwhelm mental health systems and coping strategies (Evans et al., 2017).

Psychological resilience theory is often used to explain mental health and stressful situations. It may also be observed, quantified, or explored as a trait, process, or outcome. Researchers and policy makers exploring impacts of the COVID-19 pandemic on underserved populations and under resourced locations throughout the world are using resiliency theory to explore resilience and mental health. Li and colleagues surveyed 23,192 people between the ages of 18 and 85. They found that older adult mental health was better than other age groups during the COVID-19 pandemic. Their research also found that only high levels of social support can moderate low levels of resilience in all age groups (Li et al., 2021).

Sociorelational theory advocates for ethical treatment and public health prevention policies that recognizes addiction is not an individual problem, it is a problem that results from sociorelational processes (van der Eijk & Uusitalo, 2016). Proponents of sociorelational theory call for shared responsibility and support for SUD rather than isolating individuals with shame, guilt, and judgment. This theory challenges the brain disease theories of addiction, mainly because they do not include the social and relational processes that influence brain processes before drug use. Similarly, authors criticize choice theories because the decision making process in addiction goes beyond individual choice, choices are influenced by broader social, cultural, political, and systems conditions.

Queer theory utilizes methods and strategies that bring to light an individual's identity and seeks to unpack gender as a binary concept (Kelley, 2020). Queer theorists bring out voices of the oppressed through cultural engagement, advocacy, policy, and deconstruction of dominant theories (Kelley, 2020).

Intersectionality theory can help conceptualize a person, group of people, or social problem based on discrimination and disadvantage and multiple streams of oppression, for example race, class, gender identity, sexual orientation, religion, and other identity markers (Collins, 2019; Kelley, 2020).

Multisystemic frameworks for mental health focus on recovery and resilience while targeting mental health, social cohesion, and sustainable livelihoods. Authors Lordos and colleagues applied this framework to explore what societal healing in Rwanda would and could look like after multiple human rights violations and complete devastation from genocide against the Tutsi (2021). Drawing on qualitative research approaches, authors used a grounded theory approach (to be discussed in Chapter 5) to create a conceptual taxonomy of innovations to support multi system recovery and resilience in post-genocide Rwanda. Study authors report the need for sophisticated mental health sectors, socio therapy as a hybrid intervention to address psychological trauma, reconciliation initiatives, reintegration of convicted genocide perpetrators, and ongoing efforts to address trauma (Lordos et al., 2021). With the review of evidence and theories behind us, let's discuss the differences and similarities in research and evaluation.

Public Health Takeaway- Multiple theories and frameworks guide treatment program evaluations. A public health approach requires evaluators to select theories that elevate the voices of historically marginalized and minority groups while advocating for systems change that address structural and institutional factors that perpetuate health inequities, oppressive practices, and racism.

Research and Evaluation

If you are reading this book, you might be a researcher. You might also be an evaluator, professor, student, teacher, clinician … you might be anyone. Exciting. When I meet people, they want to talk about research. I am like most researchers, thrilled to talk nonstop for hours about the people, places, interventions, findings, and meaning. Some of my research involves topics that people don't want to know about. For example, policies related to problematic sexual behavior of youth or the effectiveness of addiction treatment programs and relapse rates. These topics make some people uncomfortable. Automatically the conversation goes from thinking about research in a lab, with a rat, to major social awkwardness.

When people find out I work as an evaluator, this also sparks a curiosity... an evaluator of what and why. Similar to the discussion on research, I tend to get way too excited and talk about the evaluation of treatment programs, the need for employment programs to address social determinants of health, the requirement that evaluators advocate for social justice and change ... rather than more traditional approaches. I realize there is just a fraction of the population that cares about evaluation of treatment programs and what we are learning through our evaluations, and that is okay. People may not care about the process of evaluation, but they certainly care about what is effective, what will help and heal themselves or their loved ones who may be struggling with a MHSUD.

I would like to bring your attention to the overlaps in research in evaluation and evaluation in research. You might know or see the overlaps already in this text. For example, why explore research on MHSUD, why not review evaluations of MHSUD programs? Evaluation uses research findings and research uses evaluation. What distinguishes research from evaluation is its intended use. **Research** is about testing a theory, generalizing findings, or exploring a phenomenon for the purposes of building new knowledge or evidence. **Evaluation** on the other hand is about finding value and meaning. As evaluators we may conduct research, and as researchers we may evaluate. Table 2.3 outlines key differences between research and evaluation.

Thoughts about Research and Evaluation

Doctoral student Dana Wanzer wrote about differences in research and evaluation in a recent American Evaluation Association (AEA) blog post. She wanted to know how evaluators and researchers defined program evaluation and

Table 2.3 Research vs. Evaluation

Research	Evaluation
Produces generalizable knowledge	Judges merit or worth
Utilizes scientific inquiry based on intellectual curiosity	Utilizes program interests of stakeholder's first
Advances knowledge and theory	Provides information that is used to inform program decision-making
Takes place in a controlled setting	Takes place in various places, with different people, resources, needs, and timelines
Results are published	Results are reported to stakeholders, results may be published

differentiated evaluation from research (Wanzer, 2019). Wanzer surveyed 522 participants and found that evaluators and researchers define evaluation similar to the definite provided in this text, to determine merit, significance, or worth of something coming to a value judgment (2019). A key distinction though was that evaluators felt that evaluation was about learning, informing decision making, and improving programs, researchers did not. Half of the survey respondents felt that evaluation and research overlap, equally. A third of respondents felt that evaluation is a subcomponent of research. Respondents agreed that a key distinction between research and evaluation is the purpose, audience, recommendations, disseminating results, study design, methods, and analyses. In sum, research and evaluation are similar but different. Research aims to add knowledge to the field. Evaluation aims to make decisions or judgments about program effectiveness. While beyond the scope of this chapter and text, Wanzer's research and evaluator/researcher perspectives on purpose and differences will come up at some point in the evaluation of treatment programs- be ready to discuss and defend your approaches and purpose.

Organizations Leading Treatment Research and Evaluation

The **National Institute on Drug Abuse (NIDA)** is the leading federal agency in the United States that supports scientific research on drug use and its consequences (https://www.drugabuse.gov/). NIDA's fiscal year 2020 budget was $1.2 billion in 2020, supporting research training, research centers, research project grants, and other contracts and research.

The **National Institutes on Mental Health (NIMH)** is the leading federal agency in the United States that supports research on mental disorders (https://www.nimh.nih.gov/). NIMH's fiscal year 2020 budget was $76.4 million. Similar to NIDA, NIMH budgets support various research endeavors at the university, state, and local level. Despite increasing demands for research that addresses increases in MHSUD, both NIDA and NIMH budgets were reduced in 2020.

The **Substance Abuse and Mental Health Services Administration (SAMHSA)** (https://www.hhs.gov/sites/default/files/fy-2020-budget-in-brief.pdf) is one of the primary leaders in MHSU programming in the US. SAMHSA supports programming, pilot initiatives, prevention, and follow-up ... but they do not fund research. SAMHSA's fiscal year 2020 budget was $5.5 billion. Public and philanthropic organizations fund research.

Research on MHSUD globally is more nuanced, with different approaches to prevention, treatment, and follow-up documented, there are a number of agencies and private foundations that fund MHSUD research. A 2016 systematic review of health research funding organizations identified the top 10 funding organizations in the world, funding more than $37.1 billion (Viergever & Hendriks, 2016) which constitutes 40% of all public and philanthropic health research spending globally. The largest funder was the United States National Institutes of Health ($26.1 billion), followed by the European Commission ($3.7 billion), and the United Kingdom Medical Research Council ($1.3 billion). The largest philanthropic funder was the Welcome Trust ($909.1 million), the largest funder of health research through official development assistance was USAID ($186.4 million), and the largest multilateral funder was the World Health Organization ($135.0 million) (Viergever & Hendriks, 2016).

Gaps and Challenges in Current MHSUD Research and Evaluation

We know that the burden of MHSUD is increasing worldwide (Whiteford et al., 2013). Current research gaps are influenced by poverty, politics, poor health systems, and co-morbidities that contribute to increasing health burdens. Baingana and colleagues identified global research challenges and opportunities in their 2015 article, "Global research challenges and opportunities for mental health and substance use disorders." They identified priorities for future research and describe current gaps and challenges at the global level (Baingana et al., 2015). **Treatment gap** research is necessary because people need treatment but do not receive it in low to middle income countries (LMICs) (Baingana et al., 2015). There is a **scientific knowledge gap** about how to prevent, intervene, treat, and provide follow-up for individuals with MHSUD in LMICs. Most research is conducted in high-income countries and the utility and application of research findings is limited when applied to low-income countries. Implementation research is needed to explore MHSUD research in LMICs. Epidemiological research is necessary to explore differences in risk and protective factors in different contexts and countries. Health delivery and implementation research calls for expanding access to high quality care for LMICs using models that leverage limited clinical resources. Translational and health policy research supports evidence-based public health policy that is not well understood at the local or global level. Ongoing collaboration between researchers, policy makers, communities, institutions, and advocates are necessary to translate MHSUD research into practice and policy uptake.

Research and Evaluation Informs Social Justice and Advocacy Efforts

Research is essential because it tells us what happened, where we are at, or even where we need to go. Research can be used to inform social justice and advocacy efforts, and to redirect programs, policies, and treatment modalities to promote equity and equality. As demonstrated in the previous section, there is limited research in LMICs and this is a social justice issue.

The Global Burden of Disease Study 2019 highlights health risks from 204 countries from 1990 to 2019. Data indicate that drug use increased during this time period, and the United States has the largest increase in deaths due to drugs when compared with any other country (Institute for Health Metrics and Evaluation, 2020). Check out the resources section at the end of this chapter for more information about the study and data available. (Figure 2.3)

Number of deaths from substance use disorders, United States, 1990 to 2017

Substance use disorders refers to direct deaths from drug overdoses. This is distinguished from substance use as risk factor for premature death, which results when alcohol or drug use increases the likelihood of the development of disease or injury.

Substances shown in red are collectively termed 'Illicit drug use' in addition to cannabis, which is not shown here since it is not attributed to direct deaths from usage.

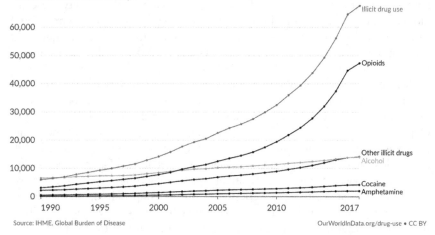

Source: IHME, Global Burden of Disease   OurWorldInData.org/drug-use • CC BY

Figure 2.3 Deaths Due to Drug Use in the United States 1990 to 2017.

(Source: IHME Global Burden of Disease, 2020).

Racial Equity

Research on **racial equity in treatment** settings is needed. Black people and Hispanics are less likely than whites to complete treatment. Researchers report the primary reason for non-completion is related to differences in **socio-economic status**, with unemployment and housing instability being the major contributing factors (Saloner & Cook, 2013). Burlew and colleagues call for funders to promote research that addresses racial and ethnic disparities to SUD treatment while increasing access to training opportunities for racial and ethnic minorities researchers. Burlew identified the following best research practices to promote racial equity: 1) ensure adequate recruitment of racial/ethnic minorities in research, 2) address central components of valid analysis, and 3) utilize adequate methods for assessing effect sizes for racial/ethnic minorities. Researchers call for a greater focus on urgent public health substance use treatment issues affecting racial/ethnic minorities and increasing the number of underrepresented racial/ethnic treatment researchers. Decision making and funding around treatment research should include racial/ethnic minority investigators. Proponents of these best practices believe that including racial/ethnic minorities in funded studies will result in new evidence and knowledge about treatment outcomes for specific racial/ethnic groups (Burlew et al., 2021).

Research and Evaluation that Equalizes Power, Increases Access, and Promotes Equity

One of the goals of public health is to integrate aspects of social justice and health equity in all aspects of evaluation and programming. I realize the importance of shared definitions, so here are two. **Social justice** is a state in which equity, fairness, opportunity and success for all diverse members of a society are commonplace and expected, in which there is acknowledgement that personal and structural success and struggles in society are intertwined, and that inequities of the past are acknowledged and redressed (Barker, 2003). **Health equity** means that everyone has a fair and just opportunity to be as healthy as possible. A healthy equity approach requires professionals to address systemic issues like poverty, discrimination, and related consequences (Braveman, 2006). If these terms are new to you, or if you just want more context check out the Five Faces of Oppression by Iris Marion Young (2011). This chapter is a cornerstone of my teachings in public health and a must read for anyone working in public health and evaluating treatment programs (Young, 2011). The Five Faces of Oppression show up everywhere, including treatment program settings. These include exploitation, marginalization, powerlessness, cultural imperialism, and violence. Young's article is a springboard for thinking about our work as evaluators and how to promote social justice and equity. Nissen, a social justice treatment program advocate, urges professionals to embrace a social justice lens and develop interventions informed by social justice principles. What does this mean? First we must address oppression and anti-oppressive practices through our work with individuals, families, communities, and polices (Nissen, 2014; Young, 2011). Here are some explorative questions that treatment programs and evaluators may use to critically examine social justice and equity (Nissen, 2014).

Work with Communities

- To what degree does the program address the economic and health disparities that relate to addiction?
- Does the community have a voice in the design, function, operation and overall measurement of success of the program?
- Are community's efforts acknowledged to create comprehensive systems and networks?

Work with Organizations

- To what degree does the treatment program challenge themselves to address diversity-related disparities in treatment access and outcomes?
- Does the organizational mission reflect social and social justice levers for action, engagement and improvement?
- Does the organization create meaningful learning opportunities for treatment practitioners to explore their own biases, stereotypes and blind spots

regarding the causes and progression of addictive behavior, as well as the possibilities of success for recovery among diverse populations?

- Does the treatment organization recruit, hire and promote diverse staff to reflect the diversity of the population served?
- Do the governing structures represent diversity within the community?

Work with Policy

- Does the treatment program actively participate in efforts to better address the policy drivers that limit and/or control access and/or availability of treatment for vulnerable and marginalized communities?
- Does the treatment program partner with communities to build better prevention and early intervention opportunities?
- How does the treatment program focus on community wellness as a policy driver for greater economic justice, school success, health and overall well-being indicators for vulnerable populations?

Work with Individuals and Families

- To what degree are program efforts with individuals and families connected to the challenges they experience in the real worlds they inhabit?
- Are poverty, houselessness, other health challenges, and other human rights concerns intersecting with the need for addictions treatment? How does the treatment program address these needs?
- Does the program acknowledge diversity in the offering, delivery, and creation of recovery support services?
- Is client voice and empowerment/strengths evident in how services are provided? (Nissen, 2014).

Public Health Takeaway- Evaluators must work at all levels to equalize power, access, and promote equity. Work with individuals, families, communities, organizations, and policies to promote health for all.

CRT mentioned earlier provides a frame for exploring issues of equity, racism, power, and social justice. There are numerous ways that researchers and evaluators can advocate for equity and justice in their work. Here are just two examples of approaches that promote equity.

Participatory evaluation and research methods represent a relatively new paradigm that connects social sciences and health care to advocacy and equity. In the last two decades, the term **community-based participatory research** (CBPR) has been increasingly used in health-related disciplines to link research, action, and education (Kelley, 2013). One note on community. Community is not just a physical location or a zip code. **Community** is a unit of identity and may represent a group of people with shared connections, common values, norms, shared interests, or priorities. One example of a community is a group of individuals participating in an out-patient treatment program.

Collectively these individuals represent a community with shared values, experiences, ideas, and access to power that makes them unique.

CBPR levels power by respecting and engaging with community. Israel and colleagues identified nine principles of CBPR that promote co-learning, capacity building, sustainability, and community benefits (Israel et al., 2013).

- Acknowledging the community as a unit of identity
- Building on the strengths and resources of the community.
- Facilitating a collaborative, equitable partnership in all phases of research.
- Fostering co-learning and capacity building among all partners.
- Achieving a balance between generating new knowledge and developing an intervention, both should be for the mutual benefit of all partners.
- Focusing the local relevance of public health problems and ecological perspectives on multiple factors that determine health.
- Involving systems development using a cyclical and iterative process, whereby the system is continuously developed in a repetitive manner to reach the desired goal or outcome of the system.
- Disseminating results to all partners and involving them in the wider dissemination of results.
- Involving a long-term process and commitment to sustainable research projects.

A **Social Determinants of Health (SDOH)** focused evaluation is useful for advancing equity and justice. WHO's SDOH framework combines psychosocial approaches, social produce of disease/policy economy of health, and eco-social frameworks to understand the main pathways of health (Kelley, 2020; Solar & Irwin, 2010). This framework is based on social context, social stratification, differential exposure, differential vulnerability, and differential consequences of health. Public health professionals and advocates utilize this evaluation framework because it addresses multiple factors that impact equity in health and well-being. Here are some attributes of the framework.

- Social economic and political context include governance, macroeconomic policies, social policies, public policies, culture and society values.
- Socioeconomic position includes social class, gender, ethnicity (racism), education, occupation, and income. One's socioeconomic position is linked to social cohesion and social capital.
- Intermediary determinants of the SDOH are material circumstances, behaviors and biological factors, and psychosocial factors. These are influenced bidirectionally by the health system.
- Combined these determinants impact equity, health and wellbeing of populations (Kelley, 2020).

Wrap Up

Wow. Research and evaluation all in one chapter. This is a lot to take in. I do not expect you to remember everything but remember some key points that we covered. These will help you as a treatment program evaluator. Early in this chapter we reviewed the socioecological model and structures, practices, and norms that may influence how treatment programs are implemented, and therefore how research, theories, and evaluation happens. Treatment programs utilize evidence-based practices, practice-based evidence, and all diverse types of evidence to inform practice and service delivery. Systematic studies from the Cochrane Review help us understand, on a large scale, what constitutes effective treatment programming. Social justice issues, health equity, racial equity, and opportunities must be a priority for all. If we are going to close the treatment gap, the scientific knowledge gap, and the health equity gap, we must begin thinking about how to create conditions that support equity, equality, and health for underserved populations in our world.

Discussion Questions

1. What are some differences between research and evaluation?
2. List three theories used in treatment settings.
3. What is the difference between evidence-based practice and practice-based evidence?
4. What is the Cochrane review? How might you use this as an evaluator?

Additional Resources

Data
Global Burden of Disease 2019 Resources, http://www.healthdata.org/
US Surgeon General's Report on Alcohol, Drugs, and Health,
https://addiction.surgeongeneral.gov/key-findings/recovery
Evidence-Based Practices
Centers for Disease Control Public Health Professional Gateway Evidence-Based
    Practices, https://www.cdc.gov/publichealthgateway/program/resources/evidence.
    html
Institute of Medicine Roundtable on Evidence-Based Medicine
https://www.cdc.gov/publichealthgateway/program/resources/evidence.html
SAMHSA Evidence-based Practices Resources Center
https://www.samhsa.gov/resource-search/ebp
Evaluation
Better Evaluation Theory of Change
https://www.betterevaluation.org/en/resources/guide/theory_of_change

References

Ajzen, I. (1991). *The theory of planned behavior. 50*(2), 179–211.

Alexander, B. K., Beyerstein, B. L., Hadaway, P. F., & Coambs, R. B. (1981). Effect of early and later colony housing on oral ingestion of morphine in rats. *Pharmacology Biochemistry and Behavior, 15*(4), 571–576. 10.1016/0091-3057(81)90211-2

Alexander, B. K., Coambs, R. B., & Hadaway, P. F. (1978). The effect of housing and gender on morphine self-administration in rats. *Psychopharmacology, 58*(2), 175–179. 10.1007/BF00426903

Baingana, F., al'Absi, M., Becker, A. E., & Pringle, B. (2015). Global research challenges and opportunities for mental health and substance-use disorders. *Nature, 527*(7578), S172–S177. 10.1038/nature16032

Ballard, P. J., Pankratz, M., Wagoner, K. G., Cornacchione Ross, J., Rhodes, S. D., Azagba, S., Song, E. Y., & Wolfson, M. (2021). Changing course: Supporting a shift to environmental strategies in a state prevention system. *Substance Abuse Treatment, Prevention, and Policy, 16*(1), 7. 10.1186/s13011-020-00341-y

Barker, R. L. (2003). *The social work dictionary.* NASW Press.

Beck Institute (n.d.) *The Home of Cognitive Behavior Therapy.* Beck Institute. Retrieved August 13, 2021, from https://beckinstitute.org/

Bell, S., Carter, A., Gartner, C., Lucke, J., & Hall, W. (2014). *Views of addiction neuroscientists and clinicians on the clinical impact of a 'brain disease model of addiction', 7*(1), 19–27.

Best, D., Gow, J., Taylor, A., Knox, A., & White, W. (2011). Recovery from heroin or alcohol dependence: A qualitative account of the recovery experience in Glasgow. *Journal of Drug Issues, 41*(3), 359–377. 10.1177/002204261104100303

Bluett, E. J., Homan, K. J., Morrison, K. L., Levin, M. E., & Twohig, M. P. (2014). Acceptance and commitment therapy for anxiety and OCD spectrum disorders: An empirical review. *Journal of Anxiety Disorders, 28*(6), 612–624. 10.1016/j.janxdis.2014.06.008

Braveman, P. (2006). Health disparities and health equity: Concepts and measurement. *Annual Review of Public Health, 27*(1), 167–194. 10.1146/annurev.publhealth.27.021405.102103

Bronfenbrenner, U. (1979). *The ecology of human development: Experiments by nature and design.* Harvard University Press.

Burlew, K., McCuistian, C., & Szapocznik, J. (2021). Racial/ethnic equity in substance use treatment research: The way forward. *Addiction Science & Clinical Practice, 16*(1), 50. 10.1186/s13722-021-00256-4

Collins, P. H. (2019). Intersectionality as critical social theory. In *Intersectionality as Critical Social Theory.* Duke University Press. 10.1515/9781478007098

Comstock, D., Hammer, T., Strentzsch, J., & Cannon, K. (2011). Relational-cultural theory: A framework for bridging relational, multicultural, and social justice competencies. *Journal of Counseling and Development—Wiley Online Library, 86*(3), 279–287. 10.1002/j.1556-6678.2008.tb00510.x

Curry, J. F., Wells, K. C., Lochman, J. E., Craighead, W. E., & Nagy, P. D. (2003). Cognitive-behavioral intervention for depressed, substance-abusing adolescents: Development and pilot testing. *Journal of the American Academy of Child & Adolescent Psychiatry, 42*(6), 656–665. 10.1097/01.CHI.0000046861.56865.6C

Delgado, R., Stefancic, J., & Harris, A. (2017). *Critical race theory (third edition): An introduction*. New York University Press. http://ebookcentral.proquest.com/lib/uncg/detail.action?docID=4714300

Engel, G. (1980). *The clinical application of the biopsychosocial model. 137*(5), 535–544.

English, D., Rendina, H. J., & Parsons, J. T. (2018). The effects of intersecting stigma: A longitudinal examination of minority stress, mental health, and substance use among Black, Latino, and multiracial gay and bisexual men. *Psychology of Violence, 8*(6), 669–679. 10.1037/vio0000218

Evans, S. Y., Bell, K., Burton, N. K., & Blount, L. G. (2017). *Black Womenas Mental Health: Balancing Strength and Vulnerability*. State University of New York Press. http://ebookcentral.proquest.com/lib/uncg/detail.action?docID=4871495

Faggiano, F., Minozzi, S., Versino, E., & Buscemi, D. (2014). Universal school-based prevention for illicit drug use. *Cochrane Database of Systematic Reviews, 12*. 10.1002/14651858.CD003020.pub3

Flynn, D., Joyce, M., Spillane, A., Wrigley, C., Corcoran, P., Hayes, A., Flynn, M., Wyse, D., Corkery, B., & Mooney, B. (2019). Does an adapted dialectical behaviour therapy skills training programme result in positive outcomes for participants with a dual diagnosis? A mixed methods study. *Addiction Science & Clinical Practice, 14*(1), 28. 10.1186/s13722-019-0156-2

Fornili, K. S. (2018). Racialized mass incarceration and the war on drugs: A critical race theory appraisal. *Journal of Addictions Nursing, 29*(1), 65–72. 10.1097/JAN.0000000000000215

Fortuna, L. R., Porche, M. V., & Padilla, A. (2018). A treatment development study of a cognitive and mindfulness-based therapy for adolescents with co-occurring post-traumatic stress and substance use disorder. *Psychology and Psychotherapy: Theory, Research and Practice, 91*(1), 42–62. 10.1111/papt.12143

Puddy, R. W. & Wilkins, N. (2011). Understanding Evidence Part 1: Best Available Research Evidence. A Guide to the Continuum of Evidence of Effectiveness. Atlanta, GA: Centers for Disease Control and Prevention. https://www.cdc.gov/violenceprevention/pdf/understanding_evidence-a.pdf

Gage, S. H., & Sumnall, H. R. (2019). Rat park: How a rat paradise changed the narrative of addiction. *Addiction, 114*(5), 917–922. 10.1111/add.14481

Government Accounting Office (n.d.) *Gao-15–405.pdf*. (n.d.). Retrieved August 13, 2021, from https://www.gao.gov/assets/gao-15–405.pdf

Gates, P., Sabioni, P., Copeland, J., Le Foll, B., & Gowing, L. (2016). *Psychosocial interventions for cannabis use disorder.* 10.1002/14651858.CD005336.pub4

Glasgow, R. E., Vogt, T. M., & Boles, S. M. (1999). Evaluating the public health impact of health promotion interventions: The RE-AIM framework. *American Journal of Public Health, 89*(9), 1322–1327. https://www.ncbi.nlm.nih.gov/pmc/articles/PMC1508772/

Grant, S., Colaiaco, B., Motala, A., Shanman, R., Booth, M., Sorbero, M., & Hempel, S. (2017). Mindfulness-based relapse prevention for substance use disorders: A systematic review and meta-analysis. *Journal of Addiction Medicine, 11*(5), 386–396. 10.1097/ADM.0000000000000338

Hasin, D. S., Saha, T. D., Kerridge, B. T., Goldstein, R. B., Chou, S. P., Zhang, H., Jung, J., Pickering, R. P., Ruan, W. J., Smith, S. M., Huang, B., & Grant, B. F. (2015). Prevalence of marijuana use disorders in the United States Between 2001–2002 and 2012–2013. *JAMA Psychiatry, 72*(12), 1235–1242. 10.1001/jamapsychiatry.2015.1858

Hoagwood, K., & Johnson, J. (2003). School psychology: A public health framework. *Journal of School Psychology, 41*(1), 3–21. 10.1016/S0022-4405(02)00141-3

Institute for Health Metrics and Evaluation. (2020). *Global burden of 87 risk factors in 204 countries and territories, 1990–2019: A systematic analysis for the Global Burden of Disease Study 2019.* (2020, October 14). http://www.healthdata.org/research-article/global-burden-87-risk-factors-204-countries-and-territories-1990%E2%80%932019-systematic

Israel, B. A., Eng, E., Schulz, A. J., & Parker, E. A.(2013). *Introduction to methods for CBPR for health (No. 4–42).* San Francisco, CA: Jossey-Bass

Jason, L. A., Guerrero, M., Lynch, G., Stevens, E., Salomon-Amend, M., & Light, J. M. (2020). Recovery home networks as social capital. *Journal of Community Psychology, 48*(3), 645–657. 10.1002/jcop.22277

Katrakazas, P., Grigoriadou, A., & Koutsouris, D. (2020). Applying a general systems theory framework in mental health treatment pathways: The case of the Hellenic Center of Mental Health and Research. *International Journal of Mental Health Systems, 14*(1), 67. 10.1186/s13033-020-00398-z

Kelley, A. (2013). Critical reflections from a community-based participatory research course. *Education for Health, 26*(3), 178. 10.4103/1357-6283.125996

Kelley, A. (2020). *Public health evaluation and the social determinants of health* (Vol. 1–1 online resource (xi, 178 pages): illustrations, maps.). Routledge, Taylor & Francis Group. https://www.taylorfrancis.com/books/9781003047810

Kelley, A., Witzel, M., & Fatupaito, B. (2017). A review of tribal best practices in substance abuse prevention. *Journal of Ethnicity in Substance Abuse, 18*, 1–14. 10.1080/15332640.2017.1378952

Kelly, J. F., Humphreys, K., & Ferri, M. (2020). Alcoholics Anonymous and other 12-step programs for alcohol use disorder. *The Cochrane Database of Systematic Reviews, 3*, CD012880. 10.1002/14651858.CD012880.pub2

Klimas, J., Fairgrieve, C., Tobin, H., Field, C.-A., O'Gorman, C. S., Glynn, L. G., Keenan, E., Saunders, J., Bury, G., Dunne, C., & Cullen, W. (2018). Psychosocial interventions to reduce alcohol consumption in concurrent problem alcohol and illicit drug users. *Cochrane Database of Systematic Reviews, 12*. 10.1002/14651858.CD009269.pub4

Kothgassner, O. D., Goreis, A., Robinson, K., Huscsava, M. M., Schmahl, C., & Plener, P. L. (2021). Efficacy of dialectical behavior therapy for adolescent self-harm and suicidal ideation: A systematic review and meta-analysis. *Psychological Medicine, 51*(7), 1057–1067. 10.1017/S0033291721001355

Lewis, M. (2015). *The biology of desire: Why addiction is not a disease.* Hachette UK.

Li, F., Luo, S., Mu, W., Li, Y., Ye, L., Zheng, X., Xu, B., Ding, Y., Ling, P., Zhou, M., & Chen, X. (2021). Effects of sources of social support and resilience on the mental health of different age groups during the COVID-19 pandemic. *BMC Psychiatry, 21*, 16. 10.1186/s12888-020-03012-1

Liddle, H. A., Dakof, G. A., Rowe, C. L., Henderson, C., Greenbaum, P., Wang, W., & Alberga, L. (2018). Multidimensional family therapy as a community-based alternative to residential treatment for adolescents with substance use and co-occurring mental health disorders. *Journal of Substance Abuse Treatment, 90*, 47–56. 10.1016/j.jsat.2018.04.011

Lordos, A., Ioannou, M., Rutembesa, E., Christoforou, S., Anastasiou, E., & Björgvinsson, T. (2021). Societal healing in Rwanda. *Health and Human Rights, 23*(1), 105–118. https://www.ncbi.nlm.nih.gov/pmc/articles/PMC8233024/

Mauer, M. (2016). *Race to incarcerate: The causes and consequences of mass incarceration.* 26. https://docs.rwu.edu/cgi/viewcontent.cgi?article=1596&context=rwu_LR

McNab, S., & Partridge, K. (2014). *Creative positions in adult mental health: Outside in-inside out.* Taylor & Francis Group. http://ebookcentral.proquest.com/lib/uncg/detail.action?docID=1660322

Mereish, E. H., & Poteat, V. P. (2015). The conditions under which growth-fostering relationships promote resilience and alleviate psychological distress among sexual minorities: Applications of relational cultural theory. *Psychology of Sexual Orientation and Gender Diversity, 2*(3), 339–344. 10.1037/sgd0000121

Meyer, I. H. (2003). Prejudice, social stress, and mental health in lesbian, gay, and bisexual populations: Conceptual issues and research evidence. *Psychological Bulletin, 129*(5), 674–697. 10.1037/0033-2909.129.5.674

Michie, S., van Stralen, M. M., & West, R. (2011). The behaviour change wheel: A new method for characterising and designing behaviour change interventions. *Implementation Science: IS, 6,* 42. 10.1186/1748-5908-6-42

Moore, G. F., & Evans, R. E. (2017). What theory, for whom and in which context? Reflections on the application of theory in the development and evaluation of complex population health interventions. *SSM - Population Health, 3,* 132–135. 10.1016/j.ssmph.2016.12.005

Nissen, L. (2014). Strengthening a social justice lens for addictions practice: Exploration, reflections, possibilities and a challenge to our shared work to promote recovery among the most vulnerable. *ATTC Messenger.* https://pdxscholar.library.pdx.edu/socwork_fac/171

Pacheco, C. M., Daley, S. M., Brown, T., Filippi, M., Greiner, K. A., & Daley, C. M. (2013). Moving Forward: Breaking the Cycle of Mistrust Between American Indians and Researchers. *American Journal of Public Health, 103*(12), 2152–2159. https://doi.org/10.2105/AJPH.2013.301480

Pickard, H. (2017). Responsibility without blame for addiction. *Neuroethics, 10*(1), 169–180. 10.1007/s12152-016-9295-2

Prochaska, J. O., & DiClemente, C. C. (1983). Stages and processes of self-change of smoking: Toward an integrative model of change. *Journal of Consulting and Clinical Psychology, 51*(3), 390–395. 10.1037/0022-006X.51.3.390

Prochaska, J. O., & Norcross, J. C. (2001). Stages of change. *Psychotherapy: Theory, Research, Practice, Training, 38*(4), 443–448. 10.1037/0033-3204.38.4.443

Saloner, B., & Cook, B. L. (2013). Blacks And Hispanics are less likely than Whites to complete addiction treatment, largely due to socioeconomic factors. *Health Affairs (Project Hope), 32*(1), 135–145. 10.1377/hlthaff.2011.0983

Substance Abuse and Mental Health Services Administration (1999). Brief Intervention and Brief Therapies for Substance Abuse. Treatment Improvement Protocol Series 34. https://store.samhsa.gov/sites/default/files/d7/priv/sma12-3952.pdf

Substance Abuse and Mental Health Services Administration & The Peter G Dodge Foundation. (n.d.) *SAMHSA's registry of evidence-based programs (NREPP) suspended.* Retrieved August 18, 2021, from https://pgdf.org/samhsas-registry-of-evidence-based-programs-nrepp-suspended/

See, N. J. (2013). Models and theories of addiction and the rehabilitation counselor. *Southern Illinois University, 34.* https://opensiuc.lib.siu.edu/cgi/viewcontent.cgi?article=1615&context=gs_rp

Solar, O., & Irwin, A. (2010). *A conceptual framework for action on the social determinants of health* (Social Determinants of Health Discussion Paper 2 (Policy and Practice)). World Health Organization. https://www.who.int/sdhconference/resources/ConceptualframeworkforactiononSDH_eng.pdf

Thoma, N., Pilecki, B., & McKay, D. (2015). Contemporary cognitive behavior therapy: A review of theory, history, and evidence. *Psychodynamic Psychiatry, 43*(3), 423–461. 10.1521/pdps.2015.43.3.423

Trauer, T. (2010). *Outcome measurement in mental health: Theory and practice.* Cambridge University Press. http://ebookcentral.proquest.com/lib/uncg/detail.action?docID=542904

US Surgeon General. (2018). *Facing Addiction in America: The Surgeon General's spotlight on opioids.* US Department of Health and Human Services. Washington, DC: HHS September 2018. https://addiction.surgeongeneral.gov/sites/default/files/Spotlight-on-Opioids_09192018.pdf

van der Eijk, Y., & Uusitalo, S. (2016). Towards a 'sociorelational' approach to conceptualizing and managing addiction. *Public Health Ethics, 9*(2), 198–207. 10.1093/phe/phw013

Viergever, R. F., & Hendriks, T. C. C. (2016). The 10 largest public and philanthropic funders of health research in the world: What they fund and how they distribute their funds. *Health Research Policy and Systems, 14*(1), 12. 10.1186/s12961-015-0074-z

Walter, K. N., & Petry, N. M. (2016). Motivation and contingency management treatments for substance use disorders. *Current Topics in Behavioral Neurosciences, 27*, 569–581. 10.1007/7854_2015_374

Wanzer, D. (2019, May 22). What is evaluation? And how does it differ from research? [American Evaluation Association]. *What Is Evaluation? And How Does It Differ from Research?* https://aea365.org/blog/what-is-evaluation-and-how-does-it-differ-from-research-by-dana-wanzer/

Whiteford, H. A., Degenhardt, L., Rehm, J., Baxter, A. J., Ferrari, A. J., Erskine, H. E., Charlson, F. J., Norman, R. E., Flaxman, A. D., Johns, N., Burstein, R., Murray, C. J. L., & Vos, T. (2013). Global burden of disease attributable to mental and substance use disorders: Findings from the Global Burden of Disease Study 2010. *Lancet (London, England), 382*(9904), 1575–1586. 10.1016/S0140-6736(13)61611-6

Wiklund Gustin, L., & Wagner, L. (2013). The butterfly effect of caring – clinical nursing teachers' understanding of self-compassion as a source to compassionate care. *Scandinavian Journal of Caring Sciences, 27*(1), 175–183. 10.1111/j.1471-6712.2012. 01033.x

Wilson, G., Farrell, D., Barron, I., Hutchins, J., Whybrow, D., & Kiernan, M. D. (2018). The use of eye-movement desensitization reprocessing (emdr) therapy in treating post-traumatic stress disorder-a systematic narrative review. *Frontiers in Psychology, 9*, 923. 10.3389/fpsyg.2018.00923

Worley, J. (2020). Therapy strategies for substance use disorders. *Journal of Psychosocial Nursing & Mental Health Services, 58*(3), 14–18. 10.3928/02793695-20200115-02

Young, I. M. (2011). *Five faces of oppression* (pp. 39–65). Princeton University Press.

3 Evaluation of Mental Health and Substance Misuse Programs

CONTENTS

DOI: 10.4324/9781003290728-3

Learning Objectives

After reading this chapter you should be able to ...

1. Summarize basic evaluation approaches used in treatment settings.
2. Describe evaluation standards established by the American Evaluation Association and Institute of Medicine.
3. List seven steps of the treatment program evaluation.
4. Differentiate the study designs used in treatment program evaluations.
5. Compare qualitative and quantitative data, and discuss analysis methods for each approach.

Introduction to Evaluation

I am many things. I am also an evaluator of mental health and substance use treatment programs. I know evaluation because I do evaluation. I am not always right, and I have made more mistakes in my work than people and clients know. However, at the end of the day, I evaluate programs because of the relentless curiosity I have about what works, for whom, why, and in what context. I want to know about value, was the investment worth the return, and did people, communities, systems, and policies benefit ... Let's begin.

A public health approach to treatment program evaluation advocates for a four-step process. A critical question that we must ask ourselves at this stage is, "What works, for whom, and when?" Evaluation includes the design and testing of prevention and treatment program approaches to determine what works (Figure 3.1).

Evaluation is about finding value. The American Evaluation Association's (AEA's) definition of evaluation is, "... a systematic process to determine merit, worth, value or significance" (American Evaluation Association, n.d.). There are many types of evaluation, product evaluation, program evaluation, policy evaluation, and personnel evaluation. This text focuses on program evaluation, used to improve effectiveness, efficiency, and results and policy evaluation, used to help policy makers assess the effectiveness of certain policies and consequences that may result from policies developed. Briefly, program evaluation questions focus on quality, outcomes, needs, conditions, variations, costs, and benefits, unintended consequences, and factors that contribute to success or lessons learned. Policy evaluation questions focus

Public Health Approach to Evaluating Substance Misuse Treatment Programs

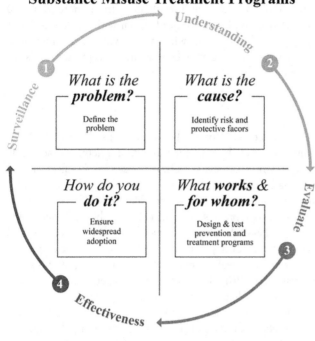

Figure 3.1 A Public Health Approach Step 3, Evaluate.

on content, implementation, and impact. Policy evaluation questions may include content articulating the goals of policy, determining if policies were implemented as planned, and if policies produced intended outcomes and impact.

Evaluation vs. evaluand. Evaluand is simply what is being evaluated. Evaluands are programs, policies, performances, products, personnel, and proposals.

Who are we? Evaluators are planners, educators, writers, program facilitators, and problem-solvers. Sometimes evaluators are viewed as judges, educators, researchers, scientists, or methodologists. Typically, evaluators have a college degree, social science research skills, strong data analysis skills (qualitative and quantitative), and professional writing abilities. Evaluators must communicate effectively, maintain professional credibility, practice effective people skills, know and observe ethical and legal requirements, navigate political issues, design, and implement evaluations, analyze, and report findings, follow-up, and manage the evaluation. Evaluators work in a variety of places. Some are employed by universities and others are based in county, city, state, or federal agencies. Private for-profit organizations and non-profit organizations employ evaluators. Evaluators also work as independent contractors and small business owners. Within treatment programs, evaluators are often external, hired by a program to assess process, outcomes, and impact.

Evaluators are everybody and anybody. There is not a licensing body for evaluators. What I do know is the American Evaluation Association (AEA) is a legitimate association of evaluators. AEA includes more than 6,000 members in 50 states throughout the United States and evaluators from more than 60 countries. AEA is not just American. If you are not familiar with AEA, check out their website and join if you want to hang with other evaluators. They have an annual conference, rad resources, a career center, and exceptional tools for evaluators https://www.eval.org/.

Four Standards

Evaluators may not have standard credentials, but evaluations do. Standards for conducting program evaluations include utility, feasibility, propriety, and accuracy. When developing and implementing an evaluation, it is essential to reflect on and answer these questions regularly. **Utility** is about who wants the evaluation and for what purpose. In treatment programs, a funding agency like SAMHSA might want an annual evaluation to demonstrate progress toward goals and objectives and use as evidence to continue funding. **Feasibility** is about practicality, time, resources, and expertise. Evaluators may want to develop a rigorous evaluation to document the effect of a treatment program, but realize there is not time, data, or resources available to support the evaluation. **Propriety** is about fairness, ethics, and, I would add, advocacy and social justice. Evaluators must consider their approach, inclusion of community, equity in funding, and addressing systems-level issues through evaluation efforts. This can be difficult because of power. I assert that a public health-focused approach advocates for evaluation contracts that include a budget-item for building and giving back to the community in a way that builds health equity and elevates social justice. We do this in my work by training Native college students from the communities that we serve in evaluation (Kelley, 2021). Students serve as evaluation interns and learn all aspects of what we do while serving their communities. Internships and training address the socioeconomic factors that are associated with MHSUD in the community by providing jobs, meaning, and purpose to students and families who may not have access to these opportunities without the evaluation contract and funding. There are other ways that propriety and justice can be achieved in evaluation. We will talk about those in Chapter 6. **Accuracy** is the last standard for evaluation, and it might be the most difficult. Accuracy ensures that findings include technically sound information that determines a treatment program's value and merit. Evaluation approaches we write in an evaluation plan change based on stakeholders' needs, contextual conditions (e.g., COVID-19 pandemic), and program implementation factors.

Public Health Takeaway—Evaluators belong to a unique discipline of professionals, with varied backgrounds, degrees, lived experiences, and positions. As advocates of a public health approach to treatment program evaluation, evaluators must understand how to elevate public health policy, standards, and health equity (step 3).

Application of Evaluation Principles Substance Misuse Treatment Settings in the United States and in the World

The AEA established a set of evaluation principles that evaluators should follow. Principles represent the core values of AEA. These principles were first developed in 1994 and updated in 2018. AEA encourages evaluators to follow these. AEA principles include systematic inquiry, competence, integrity, respect for people, and common good and equity (American Evaluation Association, 2018).

A Systematic Inquiry: Evaluators conduct data-based inquiries that are thorough, methodical, and contextually relevant.

A1 Adhere to the highest technical standards appropriate to the methods being used while attending to the evaluation's scale and available resources.

A2 Explore with primary stakeholders the limitations and strengths of the core evaluations questions and the approaches that might be used for answering those questions.

A3 Communicate methods and approaches accurately, and in sufficient detail, to allow others to understand, interpret, and critique the work.

A4 Make clear the limitations of the evaluation and its results.

A5 Discuss in contextually appropriate ways the values, assumptions, theories, methods, results, and analyses that significantly affect the evaluator's interpretations of the findings.

A6 Carefully consider the ethical implications of the use of emerging technologies in evaluation practice.

B Competence: Evaluators provide skilled professional services to stakeholders.

B1 Ensure that the evaluation team possesses the education, abilities, skills, and experiences required to complete the evaluation competently.

B2 When the most ethical option is to proceed with a commission or request outside the boundaries of the evaluation team's professional preparation and competence, clearly communicate any significant limitations to the evaluation that might result. Make every effort to supplement missing or weak competencies directly or through the assistance of others.

B3 Ensure that the evaluation team collectively possesses or seeks out the competencies necessary to work in the cultural context of the evaluation.

B4 Continually undertake relevant education, training, or supervised practice to learn new concepts, techniques, skills, and services necessary for competent evaluation practice. Ongoing professional development might include formal coursework and workshops, self-study, self-or externally-commissioned evaluations of one's own practice, and working with other evaluators to learn and refine evaluative skills expertise.

C   Integrity: Evaluators behave with honesty and transparency in order to ensure the integrity of the evaluation.

   C1   Communicate truthfully and openly with clients and relevant stakeholders concerning all aspects of the evaluation, including its limitations.

   C2   Disclose any conflicts of interest (or appearance of a conflict) prior to accepting an evaluation assignment and manage or mitigate any conflicts during the evaluation.

   C3   Record and promptly communicate any changes to the originally negotiated evaluation plans, that rationale for those changes, and the potential impacts on the evaluation's scope and results.

   C4   Assess and make explicit the stakeholders', clients', and evaluators' values, perspectives, and interests concerning the conduct and outcome of the evaluation.

   C5   Accurately and transparently represent evaluation procedures, data, and findings.

   C6   Clearly communicate, justify, and address concerns related to procedures or activities that are likely to produce misleading evaluative information or conclusions. Consult colleagues for suggestions on proper ways to proceed if concerns cannot be resolved and decline the evaluation when necessary.

   C7   Disclose all sources of financial support for an evaluation, and the source of the request for the evaluation.

D   Respect for People: Evaluators honor the dignity, well-being, and self-worth of individuals and acknowledge the influence of culture within and across groups.

   D1   Strive to gain an understanding of, and treat fairly, the range of perspectives and interests that individuals and groups bring to the evaluation, including those that are not usually included or are oppositional.

   D2   Abide by current professional ethics, standards, and regulations (including informed consent, confidentiality, and prevention of harm) pertaining to evaluation participants.

   D3   Strive to maximize the benefits and reduce unnecessary risks or harms for groups and individuals associated with the evaluation.

   D4   Ensure that those who contribute data and incur risks do so willingly, and that they have knowledge of and opportunity to obtain benefits of the evaluation.

E   Common Good and Equity: Evaluators strive to contribute to the common good and advancement of an equitable and just society.

   E1   Recognize and balance the interests of the client, other stakeholders, and the common good while also protecting the integrity of the evaluation.

   E2   Identify and make efforts to address the evaluation's potential threats to the common good especially when specific stakeholder interests conflict with the goals of a democratic, equitable, and just society.

E3 Identify and make efforts to address the evaluation's potential risks of exacerbating historic disadvantage or inequity.

E4 Promote transparency and active sharing of data and findings with the goal of equitable access to information in forms that respect people and honor promises of confidentiality.

E5 Mitigate the bias and potential power imbalances that can occur as a result of the evaluation's context. Self-assess one's own privilege and positioning within that context.

Application of AEA Principles to Treatment Program Evaluation

AEA principles hold evaluators to a high standard. These principles are all encompassing, and at times difficult to achieve. Every evaluation is unique and therefore the application of these principles to a treatment program varies. Table 3.1 highlights examples of how evaluators may apply these principles to treatment program.

The American Psychological Association (APA) developed guidelines for evaluating treatment efficacy (2002). Sometimes clinicians utilize these guidelines; in other cases, an external evaluator may follow these guidelines. APA's primary focus is based on efficacy that can be demonstrated scientifically. APA developed the following five criterion for evaluating the efficacy of MHSU interventions.

> Criterion 1.0 Guidelines should be based on broad and careful consideration of the relevant empirical literature.
> Criterion 2.0 Recommendations on specific interventions should take into consideration the level of methodological rigor and clinical sophistication of the research supporting the intervention.
> Criterion 3.0 Recommendations on specific interventions should take into consideration the treatment conditions to which the intervention has been compared.
> Criterion 4.0 Guidelines should consider available evidence regarding patient-treatment matching.
> Criterion 5.0 Guidelines should specify the outcomes the intervention is intended to produce, and evidence should be provided for each outcome (APA, 2002, p. 1054–1055).

Evaluators are most concerned with Criterion 5, outcomes of the intervention, and evidence for each intended outcome.

APA developed a list of 11 considerations for examining outcomes of treatment efficacy.

1. Participant selection
2. Treatment goals
3. Quality of life and functioning

4. Attrition
5. Long-term consequences of treatment
6. Indirect consequences of treatment
7. Patient satisfaction with treatment
8. Iatrogenic negative effects of treatment
9. Clinical significance
10. Methods
11. Treatment goals (APA, 2002, p. 1055)

Table 3.1 Select Evaluation Principles and Treatment Program Examples

Evaluation Principle	*Example*
A4. Systematic Inquiry: Make clear limitations of evaluation and it's results.	Annual evaluation report includes limitations of evaluation. Follow-up data available for only 20% of participants. Limited follow-up data decreases generalizability of evaluation and results about effectiveness.
B3. Competence: Evaluation team seeks out competencies necessary to work in the cultural context of the evaluation.	Three-person evaluation team meets with recovery program weekly, attends culture classes, visits community regularly, makes an effort to learn language, and reviews historical factors and context as they relate to MHSU and working with outsiders.
C5. Integrity: Accurately and transparently represent evaluation procedures, data, and findings.	Evaluation presents data and findings using non-technical terms and easy-to-read graphical abstracts. Evaluation represents both negative and positive outcomes related to a program. For example, intervention participants report increases in substance use despite involvement in comprehensive treatment program.
D2. Respect for People: Abide by professional ethics, standards, and regulations.	All data collected includes informed consent. Records are maintained in a locked storage cabinet and password protected dual authentication file. All data are deidentified prior to data cleaning and analysis. Intention and use of data are considered and guided by ethical standards and community/program policies.
E5. Common Good and Equity: Mitigate bias and power imbalances … self-assess privilege and position.	Evaluation team addresses power imbalance through routine self-reflection and having an equity stance. Team speaks openly about privilege and degrees earned in relation to the community and participants. Team follows a CBPR approach and principles to address power dynamics.

Treatment Program Evaluation

Treatment is often evaluated based on a specific modality, with specific populations in mind, and explored based on goals, duration, completion, and specific modalities (dual morbidities, poly drug use, relapse prevention, or aftercare services). The National Institute on Drug Abuse (NIDA) in the United States leads research and evaluation of various addiction science-related initiatives. The NIDA reports that when people get into treatment for extended periods of time, they are less likely to use drugs, less likely to be involved in criminal activity, and overall, their occupational, social, and psychological functioning improves (NIDA, 2020). The NIDA identified essential components of comprehensive drug abuse treatment programs (Figure 3.2). Any of these components could be considered as a focus for a treatment program evaluation. Boxes located in the inner circle are potential components of a treatment program evaluation.

Primary Evaluation Criteria for Treatment Clients

Before we dive into the world of evaluation, consider the difference between examining outcomes based on the individual client or outcomes related to the program. In most instances, treatment program evaluators are not working with individual-level client data but a collection of data (for example, 100 clients served by a treatment program). Treatment outcome domains that are most generally used with clients include the following four areas: (1) reduction in alcohol and drug use, (2) improved health (medical and psychiatric health, and fewer instances of emergency room visits), (3) improved social functioning (employment, family, and social relationships), and (4) improvements in healthy behaviors that translate to public health and safety (crimes and risk-taking behaviors that spread disease) (McLellan et al., 2005).

Primary Evaluation Focus Areas for Treatment Programs

Evaluating an entire treatment program is like eating an elephant, one bite at a time. Most evaluators do not eat elephants, but they may identify with the task of evaluating substantial programs. I cannot imagine all of the different evaluations that are happening as you read this chapter. The core focus of any evaluation is answering the critical evaluation question, **"How did the program/activity work?"** Treatment program evaluations may focus on an entire program (multiple trainings, prevention, screening, referral, early intervention, counseling, support, recovery, resources, staff time, activities, therapies, and modalities) or with a specific intervention, for example, Medication Assisted Treatment (MAT) for individuals with opioid use disorder (OUD) and the efficacy of MAT on treatment outcomes at three- and six-month follow up. Evaluations may also capture the numerous services provided within a treatment center and participant satisfaction, quality, relevance, and application of skills or knowledge gained.

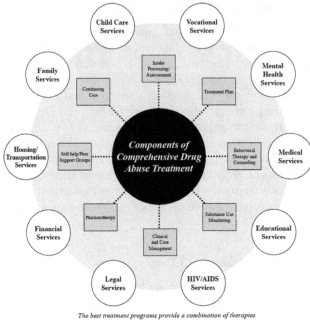

The best treatment programs provide a combination of therapies
and other services to meet the needs of the individual patients.

Figure 3.2 NIDA's Recommendations for Comprehensive Drug Abuse Treatment.

Recommended Public Health and Social Determinants Orientation

When developing a public health-oriented treatment program evaluation, it is essential to consider the social determinants of health (SDOH) (or the determinants that are taking away from health). The critical question we want to answer is, "How and why are conditions (determinants) causing (SDOH) disease (addiction) or poor health (mental, physical, emotional, spiritual)?" We will talk more about these determinants, conditions, and systems in Chapter 4–7, but for now, just trust me, they are important. As a side, I wrote an entire textbook on SDOH-focused evaluations; so, if you are wanting to do a deep dive, check it out (Kelley, 2020). In the meantime, here are six considerations to ask yourself when developing a treatment program evaluation that goes beyond the basics.

1. Is your approach holistic?
2. Did you use or consider an intersectoral approach (more than just treatment programs)?
3. Do you recognize elements of social exclusion (consider inequality, inequity, poverty, low income, and crime)?
4. Do you understand the role of individuals and communities?
5. Do you recognize the importance of upstream action (think early intervention and prevention)?

6.   Did you identify interactions between determinants or feedback loops (think systems theory)? (Kelley, 2020)

Process evaluation uses all kinds of data, including empirical data to assess the delivery of programs. **Process** can be thought of as what the treatment program is doing (interventions, activities, and trainings). **Formative evaluation** occurs when a program is being implemented with the goal of making immediate changes based on recommendations from the evaluation. Sometimes the terms formative evaluation and performance monitoring are used in evaluation (Kelley, 2018). **Performance monitoring** helps support treatment programs as they work toward their goals and implement objectives. **Performance measures** may include the number of people involved in a program or activity related to the goals of the program, the number of organizations involved, the number of individuals screened or referred, the number of people receiving services, or the number or percentage of workgroup who are part of the community or target population. Performance measures help funding agencies document outcomes associated with treatment programs and advocate for continued funding (Kelley, 2018). **Monitoring** seeks to evaluate the performance of a program or intervention (Khandker et al., 2009). Sometimes the terms monitoring and evaluation (M & E) are used in evaluation, but the purpose of monitoring compared with evaluation is different.

Impact Evaluations

Impact evaluation is used to assess the impacts of treatment programs and interventions.

Impact evaluations are characterized by innovative study designs, pilot programs, and interventions that produce solid evidence (Khandker et al., 2009). **Targets and benchmarks** are indicators used to specify a value of what is to be achieved by a given time. An example of a target is the number of recovery-oriented systems of care meetings that will occur in the first year. **Indicators** document various aspects of the program/intervention outlined in the logic model. **Indicators may include rates of participation in treatment, attitudes, behaviors, use rates, abstinence rates, short- and long-term recovery rates, and others.** An example of a specific indicator is the proportion of partners that attend at least half of the recovery-oriented systems of care meetings. **Impact indicators** measure the distal outcomes that occur over time, for example, the proportion of partners that attend at least half of the recovery-oriented systems of care meetings over a five-year period. **Impact measures** may relate to health, wellbeing, quality of life, poverty, policy, and environment. These measures are defined in the evaluation plan and used to document progress toward goals and objectives.

Outcome evaluation is similar to impact evaluation but focuses on whether a program or intervention produced the intended results. An **outcome** is the effect of the treatment program. Logic models can be helpful in conceptualizing outcomes that are both short term, intermediate, and long term. Outcome evaluations may include an assessment from the impact evaluation on each program or intervention, data from the population or group involved, and an appropriate evaluation design. When planning an outcome evaluation, it is important to identify the indicators, data, and collection strategy.

Short-term outcomes may be related to knowledge, skills, or attitudes. Short-term outcomes are generally measured immediately after the program ends. An example of a short-term outcome is a youth report increased knowledge about the dangers of binge drinking. **Intermediate outcomes** are changes in behavior or decision making that are measured after the program end. Intermediate and medium-term outcomes are usually measured several months after a program ends. An example of a medium-term outcome is a reduction in the number of underage youth who report no binge drinking in the past 30-days. **Long-term outcomes** are changes in status or life conditions. These are measured over a period of years or several years after the program or intervention has taken place. An example of a long-term outcome is reducing the binge drinking rate in underage youth in a community three to five-years after an intervention.

Implementation outcomes are another evaluation focus for treatment programs. Implementation outcomes have been defined as the program reach or spread, measured by the number of individuals served, the institutionalization or routinization or performance, and the integration of efforts into programming or systems of care. Service outcomes are based on the Institute of Medicine (IOM) standards of care and include efficiency, safety, effectiveness, equity, patient-centered focus, and timeliness. Client outcomes may include satisfaction, functioning, and symptoms related to MHSU diseases (Proctor et al., 2011). (Table 3.2)

Table 3.2 Treatment Program Implementation Outcomes

Implementation Measure	Definition in Context of Treatment Program Setting
Adoption	Intention, or initial decision, to utilize a selected approach; uptake of services
Acceptability	Perception that selected approach is agreeable or palatable to patients, providers, host medical staff, etc.; satisfaction with approach, including content, delivery, comfort level, and credibility
Appropriateness	Perceived fit, relevance, and compatibility of approach for a setting, type of provider, or patient/client
Feasibility	The extent to which approach can be conducted within a location
Fidelity	The degree to which approach was implemented as prescribed; adherence to evidence-based protocols
Implementation costs	Cost impact of implementation; marginal costs; cost effectiveness; cost–benefit
Penetration	Integration of approach within a host medical setting and related systems of care; degree of institutionalization, routinization; reach or spread
Sustainability	Degree to which services are maintained within a setting during normal, ongoing operations; continued operation after grant funding ends (if applicable)
Service provision to at-risk populations	Service volume: number and proportion of patients/clients screened; rates of delivery of recommended follow-up services
Grant compliance	Achieves selected approach service targets; rates of follow-up completion; compliance with data monitoring requirements

(Source: Adapted from Proctor et al., 2011).

General Steps for Evaluation

Here are some general steps for selecting a treatment program evaluation design informed by the public health approach to evaluation (Chapter 1). Remember, these are general steps and evaluations must adapt, reflect, uphold, and honor the unique context, culture, and norms of a given community and program.

Step 1. Create a program logic model.
Step 2. Outline and describe core activities.
Step 3. Develop critical evaluation questions.
Step 4. Select an evaluation design that meets program needs and will answer critical questions.
Step 5. Plan to collect data.
Step 6. Analyze data.
Step 7. Share results, promote equity, policy change, and elevate addiction treatment as a social justice issue.

Step 1 Logic Models

Okay this would not be an evaluation text without a logic model, right? I love logic models and I bet you do too. Let's pretend for a minute that you were just hired to conduct a treatment program evaluation. Your first step after meeting with the program and considering positionality, bias, social justice, a public health approach, and your role in the overall process is to create a logic model. Figure 3.3 is a basic program logic model for a treatment program (Kelley, 2018).

When thinking about the context and structure, consider what treatment program elements will be utilized. When thinking about the inputs and activities, these are the processes that will be explored to determine more about treatment program activities, for example, when were they delivered and to whom. Initial or short-term outcomes determine what the immediate targets of change are as a result of the treatment program. This may include knowledge, attitudes, beliefs, risk behaviors, well-being, social support, abstinence, employment, education, family reunification, or other areas. Intermediate and long-term outcomes determine what has happened because of the program or intervention, generally one to five years after implementation.

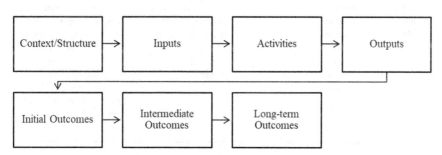

Figure 3.3 Generic Program Logic Model.

Treatment Program Logic Model

Let's see what happens to the generic logic model when we apply this framework to a treatment program and chronic pain reduction effort.

Problem: Misuse of opiates among clients with chronic pain

Local data that indicates problem: In 2020, 30% of the treatment program clients reported chronic pain and misuse of a prescription drug in the past 30-days due to chronic pain conditions. The percentage of clients with chronic pain and prescription drug misuse is higher than other treatment programs in the area. Table 3.3 outlines the use of a logic model to address a specific problem, in this case, the misuse of opiates in clients with chronic pain.

Step 2 Outline and Identify Core Activities

Once the first logic model draft is complete, it is time to think about core activities. Core activities help us answer the critical evaluation question, "How did activities work?"

Core activities include everything that is included within a program that is under evaluation, for example, processes and strategies utilized to reduce opiate use within a treatment population.

Step 3 Develop Critical Evaluation Questions

This might be the most difficult part of the treatment program evaluation planning process. Evaluators like everyone else, want to know what works. We are in the midst of the greatest addiction, mental health, and social justice crisis of our time. If

Table 3.3 Logic Model Example Opiates and Chronic Pain

Context/ Intervening Variable	Activities/ Strategy	Target Group	Outputs	Outcomes
Misuse of opiates in clients with chronic pain	Weekly alternative pain manage- ment (APM) sessions including acupunc- ture and massage	Clients with OUD	Number of clients targetedNumber of clients identified and referred to APM sessions Number of APM sessions offered by treatment program	Short-term- Increase in awareness, knowledge, attitudes, about APM sessions, reduced emergency department overdosesIntermediate- APM relieves chronic pain, perception about APM changes among clientsLong-term- Decrease in OUD, lower healthcare costs, improved physical and mental health

we know more about what aspects of a treatment program work, for whom, and when we can share the good news with the world and transform the current crisis into a state of collective well-being, justice, and equity.

It is essential to identify core elements of a treatment program that will be considered in an evaluation. With your core set of activities developed, list each activity and write how did this core activity work. Once you have listed the activities and how they work, move to the next phase of the question-building process. Link core activities to desired outcomes. For example, if a treatment program offered alternative pain management sessions for OUD, a critical evaluation question might be, "How did these sessions reduce prescription drug use?"

Step 4 Select an Evaluation Design

You have been waiting for this section for a while. You might even be a tad upset we are in Chapter 3, and just getting to the good stuff of study designs. I cannot tell you what type of study design to use in your treatment program evaluation because I am not with you. I can tell you what I know about selecting the right design. First, consider the program goals and objectives, the reasons for the evaluation, and what key stakeholders want from the evaluation. One of the most frequent evaluations I conduct of treatment programs are summative in nature, they focus on the overall quality and impact of a program, and if a selected intervention led to changes in behaviors or desired outcomes. Summative evaluations require causality, meaning, did the intervention produce the outcome, or did something else. Efficacy or pilot studies may be conducted to determine if an intervention produces the desired effect, even on a small scale. Efficacy or pilot study data can then be used to implement larger studies, in different populations to determine effectiveness. Although an evaluator's role is never just about determining causality, it is essential that evaluators conduct their work in a systematic way that creates required evidence about a program or intervention. Evaluators may conduct outcome evaluations with treatment programs. When implementing an outcome evaluation, it is essential for evaluators to consider these three questions: (1) Did the intervention begin before the changes in outcomes occurred, (2) Does the outcome remain unchanged if there is no intervention in place? (3) Can you rule out all other possible causes or contributing factors related to changes in the outcomes? (Telfair et al., 2022).

Randomized experimental evaluation designs (Figure 3.4) are the most rigorous, sought after, gold standard evaluation in the field. Randomized evaluations result in the greatest validity and make it easier for evaluators to demonstrate causality between the intervention and the desired outcome. Randomized experiments require random assignment. There are a number of ways to randomly assign participants to an intervention/treatment group or a control/non-treatment group. Evaluators (from all walks of life, programs, positions, and ideologies) use a core set of evaluation designs to guide their approach. You may know about these already, but for those who do not know, let's dive in.

Evaluation designs help evaluators determine what needs to be measured and how it will be measured. **Descriptive evaluation designs** are used to describe aspects

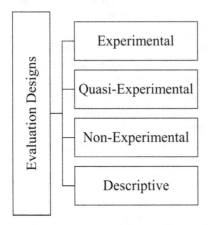

Figure 3.4 Evaluation Designs.

of a treatment program, process, outcome, or impact. For example, a descriptive evaluation design may include the types of activities implemented, who implemented them, who attended, and how activities impacted outcomes of interest.

Non-experimental designs may be descriptive, and evaluators may conduct a non-experimental evaluations for a variety of reasons. For example, lack of comparison group, limited resources, limited funding, limited time, and difficulty isolating intervention components. Non-experimental designs do not include a control or comparison group. A key requirement for a non-experimental evaluation design is for evaluators to have a clear conceptual understanding of how the intervention is meant to influence the outcomes of interest (Telfair et al., 2022).

There are **two main types of non-experimental study designs**. The first is a **time-series design** that uses pre-intervention trends to document what will happen following the introduction of the treatment program intervention in a specific population. Ideally, evaluators will utilize multiple observations of the intervention group pre- and post-intervention. Data is collected and analyzed to determine if treatment program or intervention impacted overall trends in outcomes of interest.

The second non-experimental design is a **pre-test and post-test** with a treatment or intervention group. Data collected from tests allow evaluators to explore differences from the start to finish of a treatment. Pre-test and post-test designs capture changes in outcome indicators, Box 3.1.

For a post-test only design, the observations between the intervention and comparison group are compared after the intervention and differences between the groups are assumed to be indicative of program effects (Telfair et al., 2022). Program impact is the difference between the intervention and control group after implementation ([O1-O2] +/– error).

If randomization is not possible, the **quasi-experimental design** is the next best thing. Quasi-experimental designs measure results at the treatment program and population levels. Quasi-experimental designs also demonstrate impact of a given intervention or treatment, Box 3.1.

Box 3.1   Evaluation Study Designs

Non-experimental Pre-Post-test Design

O1   X   O2   Intervention/Treatment group

X = Intervention/Treatment
O1, O2 ... O4 = Group observations at time T

Non-experimental Time Series Design

O1   O2   O3   X   O4   O5   O6   Intervention/Treatment group

X = Intervention/Treatment
O1–O6 = Group observations at time T

Quasi Experimental Design Intervention/Treatment Group

⤴   X   O1   Intervention/Treatment group
[NR]
⤵   O2   Comparison group
[NR] = Non-random assignment to groups
X = Intervention/Treatment
O1, O2 = Group observation at time T

Experimental Design

O1   X   O2   Intervention group
[R]
⤵ O3   O4   Control group
[R] = randomization
X = Intervention
O1 ... O4 = Group observation at time T

A true **experimental design** includes randomization of participants to intervention or control groups. Control groups have similar characteristics as the intervention groups, the only difference is that they did not receive the intervention. When a control group is possible, evaluators can explore the **counterfactual**, or what would have happened if the intervention or treatment did not occur. If you are planning an experimental design, collect baseline data on key indicators with both groups before the intervention occurs. After the intervention is complete, review the same key indicators and compare differences based on group status (Padian et al., 2011; Telfair et al., 2022).

During the design and planning stage it is essential to consider the **power, sample size, and effect size.** Almost all quantitative evaluations can benefit from conducting a power analysis and determining sample size before implementing an evaluation. **Sample size** refers to the ideal number of people that will be recruited (for an intervention, evaluation, study, etc.). **Power is the probability of a true positive study or evaluation finding** (or rejecting the null hypothesis) and is calculated as 1-β (also expressed as "1 - Type II error probability") (Serdar et al., 2021). Ideally, studies will have a power of 0.8 also written as 80% (Lipsey & Hurley, 2009), this means that there is an 80% chance of detecting a statistically significant difference when there is one. **Effect size** is used to determine if statistically significant differences observed are large enough to be meaningful.

If you are overwhelmed with the idea of power and sample size here are some basic rules to follow. Most statisticians agree that 100 is a solid number required to obtain meaningful results, unless the population is less than 100, then everyone within the population would need to be surveyed or included in the sample. Generally, 10% of the population is recommended for estimating the sample size, as long as this does not exceed 1,000 people. I recommend creating a sample size based on your evaluation aims, capacity, population, and resources.

Power and Sample Size Best Practices

The Abdul Latif Jameel Poverty Action Lab identified six best practices for determining sample size and statistical power. These include, (1) a larger sample increases the statistical power, (2) if the effect size is small, a larger sample is needed to achieve desired level of power, (3) evaluations with fewer clients or participants over time may need a larger sample, (4) if the population is highly variable, a larger sample is needed, (5) power is most beneficial when equally distributed between a treatment and control group, and (6) randomizing with clusters opposed to individuals reduces power (JAP-L, 2018).

There are various ways to calculate power and sample size, but G*Power is the best. It is a free online calculator for estimating power and sample size for social, behavioral, and biomedical sciences (Faul et al., 2007).

Several factors must be considered when determining sample size and this chapter does not address all considerations. Check out the Resources Section at the end of this chapter for more information on sample size calculations and power.

Step 5. Plan to Collect Data

Data that you will collect depends on the completion of Steps 1–4 presented earlier. Evaluation instruments are anything that is used in an evaluation to collect data needed for the treatment program evaluation (Kelley, 2018). Before you collect any data, consider how it will be stored, used, and protected. Confidentiality and Data use agreements (DUA) may be helpful when beginning an evaluation (see appendices for specific examples). These outline how data will be accessed, utilized, stored, and protected. Data collection approaches may include document reviews, key informant interviews, focus groups, observation, audiovisual materials, social media data, electronic health record data, or surveys. Evaluators must consider the sampling strategies they plan to use, the limitations of each strategy, and the strengths and weaknesses of each approach. Before collecting any data, develop a process for extracting, organizing and systematically tracking data that will be used in the evaluation.

Some evaluation designs will require a sampling method. The **target population** represents the entire population that is under evaluation, sometimes this is also referred to as the universe. The evaluation or **study population** includes individuals that an evaluator has access to, for example those within a treatment program. The **sampling frame** is the actual population from which the participants will be recruited for the study or evaluation. For example, clients enrolled in Level 2.0 care at a community recovery center from June 2020 to June 2021. The **sampling method** is how an evaluator will recruit or identify individuals that are part of the sampling frame.

There are two types of sampling strategies commonly used in evaluation, **probability sampling** (remember the experimental design earlier, with randomization), this is an example of probability sampling because it is based on chance events. **Non-probability sampling** is the second type of sampling used in evaluations, it involves selecting the population that is accessible and available (Setia, 2016). **Qualitative sampling** involves selecting a group of individuals based on their experiences with an issue. These individuals belong to a population of interest and give voice and meaning to a specific topic area. While beyond the scope of this text, these are some distinct types of **sampling strategies**: convenience sampling, random sampling, simple random sampling, stratified sampling, systematic sampling, cluster sampling, multistage sampling, purposive sampling, voluntary sampling, quota sampling, respondent driven sampling, qualitative sampling, and snowball sampling (Kelley, 2018, 2020; Setia, 2016).

The most common sampling strategy I use in treatment program evaluation is a **non-probability convenience sampling**. This approach is the most criticized, but the easiest to implement. In convenience sampling, evaluators select individuals based on their availability and willingness to participate in an evaluation or study. These individuals do not represent the entire universe or target population; however, a convenience sampling approach is useful in documenting overall needs, comparing treatment need and outcome data with other populations (via administrative data), developing or generating hypotheses or theories of change, and for quality improvement and reporting purposes (Kakinami & Conner, 2010). A disadvantage of convenience sampling is selection bias. I also utilize various forms of qualitative sampling including **homozygous sampling** (used to describe a small group of five to ten people with in-depth focus groups or interviews), **typical case sampling** (used to describe what is typical within a treatment program or individual experience) or **snowball sampling** (used in treatment program settings where a respondent in a sample is asked to identify others within the sample that may be willing to participate). **Qualitative sampling** has several advantages, data are rich and detailed, and provide in-depth understanding and meaning about a given phenomenon, for example understanding spiritual aspects of recovery

(Green et al., 1998). Disadvantages of qualitative sampling include selection bias, time and resources required, and results may be viewed as less than quantitative data collected via probability sampling and randomized design studies (Kakinami & Conner, 2010). Sampling adequacy in qualitative research and evaluation has been studied extensively and relates to both composition and size. Experts have not agreed on the issue of how many people need to be included in the sample. Here is what some authors say. Morse indicates that qualitative sampling sufficiency is not about a number but about the quality and usability of data (Morse, 2000). Green and Thorogood recommend interviewing 20 people (Greene, 2005). Lincoln and Guba, the qualitative research gods, call for a sample size determination based on informational redundancy (saturation), meaning that when qualitative data is collected there are no new concepts, themes, or information emerging from data collection (Lincoln & Guba, 1985). The concept of saturation is the most widely used in qualitative sampling and evaluation. Saturation originates from the field of grounded theory, a methodological approach to developing a theory based on data collection, analysis, and emerging theories and theoretical categories.

Bias is the difference between the sampling value or population and the true population. There are multiple types of bias in the evaluation of treatment programs. **Selection bias** occurs when the selection differs between respondents in the sample and results in an unrepresentative sample (Kakinami & Conner, 2010). **Information bias** is also known as misclassification and is extremely common and includes self-reporting bias, measurement error bias and confirmation (Althubaiti, 2016). **Confounding bias** occurs when linking an exposure (like attendance in a treatment program) to an outcome (like decreased use of drugs or alcohol). Evaluators may not know other treatment programs or activities happening within an individuals life that produce the same effect. For example, an individual attends weekly treatment sessions with a licensed addiction counselor (focus of the evaluation) and also attends evening Narcotics Anonymous (NA) meetings not captured within the evaluation or individuals records. Other forms of bias may occur at varying stages of the evaluation. In the planning stage, bias may occur because of a flawed study design, or selection bias. During the implementation of evaluation, bias may occur because of social desirability bias, interviewer vias, recall bias, performance bias, transfer bias (meaning), misclassification of treatment outcomes. Bias may also occur after an evaluation ends during the reporting or publication process through citation bias and confounding (Pannucci & Wilkins, 2010).

Validity ensures that an evaluation or an instrument measures what it is supposed to measure (Kelley, 2018). There are four primary types of validity used in treatment program evaluation: conclusion validity, internal validity, construct validity, and external validity. Briefly, **conclusion validity** establishes a relationship between a treatment and an outcome. **Internal validity** documents the relationship between the treatment and the outcome observed. **Construct validity**is the degree to which a test or question measures what it should measure. **External validity** is how well the findings from an evaluation can be generalized to other groups or populations (Kelley, 2020; Pannucci & Wilkins, 2010).

Lincoln and Guba established **evaluative criteria** for qualitative research (and evaluation) based on the concept of trustworthiness. **Trustworthiness** includes credibility, transferability, dependability, and confirmability. Accomplishing credibility involves engagement, observation, triangulation, peer engagement, and member checking. **Transferability** is achieved by using thick descriptions or detailed accounts of what is happening. **Dependability** occurs via inquiry audits and confirmability may be established using audits, triangulation, and reflexivity (Lincoln & Guba, 1985). For more on evaluative criteria, review the Resources Section at the end of this chapter.

Public Health Takeaway- Multiple sampling strategies exist, make sure that you are not just focused on generalization, randomization, power, and rigor. Focus on the individuals, places, and conditions in the sample that give meaning and voice to what is happening and what needs to change for equity and social justice.

Common Evaluation Measures United States and World

Evaluation measures are essential for documenting the effectiveness of programs, exploring value and impact, and tracking overall performance of treatment program efforts. One of the key challenges and criticisms is the lack of standard definitions and instruments to assess recovery or treatment outcomes (McLellan et al., 2005; Proctor et al., 2011). As you might imagine there are multiple possibilities about the types of evaluation measures to collect with treatment programs. Here are some considerations for selecting the appropriate evaluation measures and design for a given treatment program or therapeutic intervention.

- Variables used may be process or outcome focused, program, therapist, or participant variables, relationship level variables, cultural variables, change variables, or outcome variables. All require a slightly different evaluation approach to collect, analyze, and report.
- Quantitative variables are often used to track progress throughout treatment, for example, "In the last 30-days, how many days have you used methamphetamines?" The response is a number between 1 and 30.
- Qualitative approaches include conditional, contextual, or other data that cannot be easily enumerated. I tell my students that quantitative data tells us what, and qualitative data tells us why. Examples of qualitative data may include interviews, observations, or open text response feedback from participants.

Here is a list of common measures used in evaluation of treatment programs in the United States and across the world. These can be qualitative, quantitative, or both.

Demographic information. Consider race, ethnicity, age, educational attainment, current enrollment in education or job skills programs, income level, housing status, insurance status, pregnancy status, address, and other variables of interest as determined by the MHSU program (Rural Health Information Hub, n.d.).

Indicators. Indicators include variables that assess on aspects of a program or a project. In evaluation, indicators may be used to show the types of activities that are planned, and if these activities have contributed to changes in behaviors, knowledge, or skills (based on outcome evaluation focus). Experts feel that there should be at least one indicator for each aspect of a program activity outlined in a logic model. The acronym SMARTIE is a straightforward way to remember how to design and assess indicators where S = specific, M = measurable, A = achievable, R = realistic, T = timely, I = inclusive, E = equitable (Telfair et al., 2022).

Outputs. These are often quantitative or numeric results of a program activity. We recently evaluated a vocational rehabilitation program in partnership with a treatment center (the center referred individuals to the program, and the program individuals to treatment). The **activity** is the number of workforce readiness trainings that the treatment program hosted during a specific time period. The **output** is the number of people that attended the workforce readiness training sessions.

Outcome measures. These depend on the overall goals of the treatment program but focus on what happened as a result of the program. These may include rates of MHSUD in a given organization or community, hospitalization, MHSUD emergency department visits, opioid and drug overdose, binge drinking, underage drinking, underage substance use, and abstinence rates (Rural Health Information Hub, n.d.).

Outcomes and Indicators. You may be wondering what the difference is between an outcome and an indicator. As we mentioned earlier, indicators tell us if an outcome has occurred, and how by how much it occurred. Let's consider the example we used earlier. A treatment program is offering workforce readiness classes. The **outcome** of this workforce program is to increase the number of clients employed at follow-up, the **indicators** are the number of workforce training sessions attended, the number of clients employed part or full-time at follow-up, and the level of job readiness among clients.

Cost Savings as an Outcome

Some MHSU outcome evaluations focus on the cost savings of a given program or intervention. There are different approaches for calculating cost savings. Cost savings approaches are based on certain assumptions. For example, the Department of Health and Human Services (DPHHS) published a summary of the social costs of substance abuse based on lost material goods, decreased productivity, and the cost of treatment and medical services. In 1999, DPHHS reported the total annual costs of substance abuse was $510.8 billion (Cost-Benefits-Prevention, n.d.). A report published by the Recovery Centers of America in 2016 estimated the cost of substance abuse in the US at $1.45 trillion in economic and societal harms (health, product, crime, law enforcement, criminal justice, research and development, fires, public assistance, social services, and traffic collisions) ("Economic Cost of Substance Abuse in the United States, 2016," n.d.).

Cost-effectiveness analysis (CEA) is another approach used to assess the costs and health outcomes associated with one or more interventions. CEA's are essential for evaluators working in treatment settings to help determine which interventions are most cost-effective, especially when implemented on a larger scale. Examples of how CEA is operationalized in evaluation may include death or illness averted, or disability-adjusted liver years increasing as a result of a particular intervention. Fairley and colleagues assessed the cost effectiveness of OUD treatment in association with treatment outcomes in the United States (2021). Participants received the following interventions, **Medication-assisted treatment (MAT)** with buprenorphine, methadone, or injectable extended-release naltrexone; psychotherapy (beyond standard counseling); **overdose education and naloxone distribution (OEND)**; and **contingency management (CM)** (Fairley et al., 2021). Primary outcomes and measures included fatal and nonfatal overdoses and deaths over a 5-year period, discounted lifetime **quality-adjusted life-years (QALYs)**, and costs. CEA results show that when criminal justice cost and all forms of MAT (with buprenorphine, methadone, and naltrexone) were considered, the cost savings compared with no treatment was $25,000 to $105,000 in lifetime costs per person (Fairley et al., 2021). This is a lot to take in so check out this example of a CBA that we recently conducted for a treatment program evaluation.

We reviewed funding that supported prevention and treatment efforts at one location and applied the 7:1 ratio to estimate cost savings. The individual cost to support each peer was $775.00 over a 6-month period. The program conducted intakes on 206 peers. These peers received treatment from peer mentors with the lived experience of recovery. For each peer, the cost savings was $5,425.00 (this amount is based on the per unit cost of $775.00 × 7). The per unit cost savings of $5,425 was then multiplied by 206, the number of peers in the program. The total cost savings based on the 7:1 ratio for all peers is $1,117,550.

Public Health Takeaway—The costs of treatment in the United States are some of the highest in the world. Evaluators have a massive job when exploring cost savings as an outcome in evaluation. The investment of evaluation and evidence-based treatment is the path forward (steps 3–4).

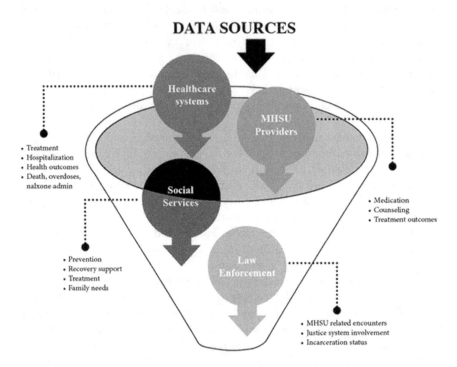

Figure 3.5 Data Collection Sources and Descriptions.

Data Collection Sources

Data may be classified as individual client-level data collected by healthcare systems, social services, or MHSU providers. Client data is often collected using validated data collection instruments such as the Addiction Severity Index (ASI), the Maudsley Addiction Profile, the Opiate Screening Assessment, or the World Health Organization Quality of Life tool. Figure 3.5 includes potential data sources and descriptions used in MHSU program evaluation.

Client level data. Evaluators may use different methods to explore effectiveness. For example, baseline data collection during intake is essential for establishing where clients are at when they start programs, and the kinds of resources they need to be successful.

Most treatment programs utilize **electronic health records (EHRs).** Clinicians utilize EHRs to conduct a variety of assessments and intakes with clients. In some cases, the clinician conducts the assessment in real time with the client responding to questions and entering data into the EHR. In other instances, clinicians use paper and pen survey tools and manually enter data later into an EHR. Examples of data collected in EHR systems include client intakes, discharge, diagnosis, scheduling, and client charts. Clinical tools include screening, assessment placements, progress notes, treatment plans, medication management, and others. EHRs provide real-time data about clients and programs using functions such as manager reports, analysis and query, and systems questionnaires.

EHR's allow you to store all client information in one location. Evaluators may access EHR's directly or work with program staff to pull data required for an evaluation.

SAMHSA is one of the major federal agencies that funds treatment programs and evaluation. Many SAMHSA funded treatment programs require use of **the Government Performance and Results Act (GPRA) tool** (see, https://www.samhsa. gov/sites/default/files/GPRA/csat_gpra_client_outcome_measures_tool_2017.pdf). The Office of Management and Budget (OMB) updates and approves the GPRA tool regularly and outlines the public reporting burden for data collection (in the case of one GPRA program tool completion time is estimated at 36 minutes). The types of questions included in the GPRA include behavioral health diagnosis, planned services, demographics, military family and deployment, drug and alcohol use, family and living conditions, education, employment, and income, crime and criminal justice status, mental health and physical health problems, treatment and recovery status, and social connectedness. Often, programs will include additional questions based on the type of program being implemented, for example a program utilizing MAT may include questions about MAT use, dose, access, and side-effects. GPRAs are collected at intake, follow-up (3, 6, and 12 months) and at discharge. programs complete a summary report with the types of services received, and any discharge information that is relevant to the client. Other evaluation data collection approaches include data collected via social media platforms like Facebook, Twitter, Instagram, mHealth interventions, eRecovery apps and programs, and more. As you might imagine there are a dozen diverse ways that programs collect data, and here are some of the most common data collection strategies used.

Facebook is a popular social media platform that many clients and programs use to engage, access groups, learn about recovery activities, or connect with other people in recovery. Some organizations have Facebook pages for specific programs. User data from Facebook can be analyzed and reported by fan demographics including age and gender. Geo-targeting on Facebook allows evaluators to assess Facebook audiences by country and city. Facebook analytics include page data, post data, and video data. Programs may track Facebook counts, impressions, engagements, and post link clicks. Evaluators may use Facebook data to explore the types of posts that are shared the most, the types of content that are most popular, along with the geographic location and demographics of frequent users. Collecting and analyzing Facebook data takes little effort and is a powerful way to explore reach, impact, needs and context of individuals, communities, and other programs.

eRecovery Data

With the present COVID-19 pandemic, many treatment programs are moving toward eRcovery and telehealth services. When collected in a systematic way

Table 3.4 eRecovery Data Collection from Smartphone Recovery App

Number of People Using the Smartphone App by Month and Week, User Type, Average Days

Screen Name	Facility Name	Page Views
JHappy	Oregon Recovery Clinic	154
Average days of Smartphone app service use by page view		
	Number of Views	Average in Past 30 Days
Sober support	780	5
Recovery tracker	330	3
Recovery resources	250	10
My motivation	800	16
My clinic	400	14
Coping with Cravings	200	29

and included in an overall evaluation plan, **eRecovery data** provides a comprehensive description of client needs, treatment effectiveness, resources utilized, and overall satisfaction with eRecovery services. There are multiple eRecovery data sources available and used by programs. CHESS Health is one company that implements eRecovery services and collects data using an app. Data in the CHESS Health Connections App includes sobriety streaks, connections, messages, planning, and discovering resources. Client data is also tracked by CHESS Health and used by evaluators. Table 3.4 is an example of eRecovery data pulled from a Smartphone app.

SMS Data

SMS includes text messaging data and evaluators may utilize SMS data to measure engagement, if the timing and dose of messages moderates or mediates outcomes, or if there is a specific threshold for engagement to realize intervention effects. Researchers have utilized various approaches to measure engagement with mobile and digital health interventions, including in-depth interviews with users, ecological momentary analysis (EMA), and reviews of system use data (Wrobel et al., 2022). In a recent evaluation of an SMS intervention to reduce suicide and drinking in youth, researchers explored the relationship between the timing of message delivery and the timing of message link clicks. Study authors reviewed clicks based on gender, message content, psychosocial health outcomes (Rushing et al., 2021).

Prevention Data

Programs often promote prevention, treatment, and follow-up services. Up until now, data collection approaches have focused mainly on client-level data. Program prevention data and processes are often collected by evaluators and SAMHSA's Strategic Prevention Framework provides one example of the categories of prevention data that programs may collect (SAMHSA, n.d.). Assessment data may include documenting needs based on data. Capacity data includes documenting local resources and readiness to change or address prevention needs identified. Planning data includes documenting what programs are doing and how they are doing it. Implementation data includes documenting how programs and practices are being delivered and how they relate to prevention. The evaluation may collect process and outcome data about the program and practices to determine if a program is successful. Outreach in community, number of people served, types of services needed, satisfaction with services, needs data, impact data, and other data. If you want more information, Chapter 5 includes examples of data collection approaches from real-world treatment program evaluations.

Service and Systems Level Data

A treatment program may collect or utilize multiple data systems to track services provided and performance improvement standards. Examples of these services and systems include quality improvement initiatives, training records for program staff, increases in capacity to provide evidence-based treatment, development of new policies and procedures or revisions to existing documents, and systems level data access and protection policies and agreements. Referral sources, referral partners, clinician hours and billable hours, overall facility follow-up rates, funding and third-party billing related data, and others as defined by a program's scope of work and need.

Qualitative Data

Qualitative data is anything that is non-numeric (Palinkas, 2014). Examples of qualitative data include observation notes, meeting minutes, focus group transcripts, photographs, narratives, journals, field notes, interview transcripts, preexisting records with qualitative data, photographs, videos, art, music, poetry (Kelley, 2018, 2020). A note on quantification, some evaluators and researchers will quantify qualitative data (called quantification). **Quantification** involves counting and manipulating (yes manipulating) qualitative data for the purpose of explaining and describing a phenomenon or answering an evaluation or research question. We will discuss the quantification of qualitative data later in this text. For now, just sit with the idea that quantification exists and is practiced widely in the treatment program evaluation milieu.

Step 6. Analyze Data

Once you have collected data it must be analyzed. Consider developing a data analysis plan before any analysis begins (Kelley, 2018). Here are some initial ideas for analyzing data. First, consider what type of data that you have (Table 3.5).

Table 3.5 Comparing Data Types

Qualitative Data	Quantitative Data
Ex. Perspectives, Impacts, Behaviors, Satisfaction	Ex. Age, Weight, Temp, Rate of Opioid Use
Describes	Quantifies
Observed	Measured
Subjective	Objective
Quality	Quantity

Quantitative Data Analysis Plan

A **data analysis plan** should include the following components.

Title. List a descriptive title of the data analysis plan.

Background. Summarize research, existing evidence, gaps in knowledge, and contextual information about the program.

Evaluation objectives. List the aims of the program as they relate to the analysis, for example, "Assess the prevalence of Adverse Childhood Experiences (ACEs) in treatment program population from 2016 to 2021." Include the evaluation study design (for example non-experimental design).

Measures. List the instrument and measures that will be used to address evaluation objectives (demographic characteristics, employment status, family status, racial or ethnic classification) and use standardized measures when possible or measures that are supported by research as it relates to your evaluation focus. For example, the 10-question ACEs instrument could be used to assess previous ACEs in treatment population (Watson, 2019).

Describe any qualitative data that will be collected in addition to standardized quantitative instruments.

Sampling. Discuss the sampling method that you will use to collect data.

Evaluation Timeline. Include a timeline for the overall program and highlight data collection or reporting dates.

Define the population. List the inclusion and exclusion criteria. For example, inclusion criteria might be written consent and 18 years or older at the time of data collection.

Data collection. Discuss when and where data collection will begin and end.

Analysis plan. Describe how data will be analyzed. For example, descriptive and multivariable analyses will be conducted to examine ACE scores of survey respondents. Survey responses will be weighted to adjust for undersampling in the population. Only responses that include responses to all questions will be included in the analysis. Chi-square testing will be used to compare the prevalence of ACEs and demographic characteristics.

Study measures and variable definitions. Include a summary of the questions, question descriptions, and value definitions. For example, for gender would be described as follows:

Column name, gender. Question number, 1. Question and or description, Which best describes your gender identity? Value definitions, 1 = male, 2 = female, 3 = transman, 4 = transwoman, 5 = genderqueer, 6 = cisgender, 7 = different identity, please describe.

Power and sample size considerations. Discuss how you will calculate power and sample size. Power and sample sizes are used to determine how many people are needed to answer an evaluation or research question (Jones, 2003). Check out the Resources Section at the end of this chapter for more on power and sample size.

Analyzing Quantitative Data

Quantitative data includes anything that is a number or that can be converted to numeric form. Earlier in this chapter we presented several examples of quantitative data that may be used in a treatment program evaluation. After you have cleaned your data, conduct simple analyses using basic **descriptive statistics** like frequencies, percentages, means, medians, modes, standard deviations, and ranges (Kelley, 2018). **Inferential statistics** may be used to explore data as it relates to the population, including differences, associations, predictions, similarities, and effects. Evaluators should refer to the total sample of a population using 'N' and a sub-group within a population is referred to as 'n' (Kelley, 2018). Descriptive data may include a mean and standard deviation. Where 'M' represents the **Mean** or the average value of a sample or population and 'SD' represents the **standard deviation** or the square root of the variance. **Variance** is the average of square differences between observations and their means (Kelley, 2018).

Statistical significance is used to document differences in an outcome due to chance. Most often significance levels are set at (p) .95. This means that there is a 95% chance that the results are true, or $1\text{-}p$. Significance is reported using (p) .001 or .05, these numbers mean there is a .001% or 5% chance the results are false. **Hypotheses testing** relates to the significance levels above and is used to test ideas about a group or population. There is a null hypothesis (H_0) and an Alternative hypothesis (H_1). The null hypothesis is a statement that we assume to be true. The Alternative hypothesis (H_1) is used when we reject the null and find the alternate hypothesis to be true. **Alpha (α)** is the lowest level that can be used to reject the null hypothesis. **Beta (β)** is the probability of a Type II error. Type 1 errors and Type II errors happen all of the time (bummer), where evaluators reject the null hypothesis, even if it is true or correct. **Cohen's d** represents the **effect size**, calculated by the mean of the intervention or treatment group minus the mean of the control or comparison group divided by the standard deviation. Cohen's d works best if you have sample that is greater than 50 (Mysiak, 2020). Although hypotheses testing and terminology are most frequently associated with research rather than evaluation, there are instances when evaluators will utilize a hypothesis testing approach to test critical evaluation questions.

Table 3.6 Evaluating Study Findings

Evaluation/Study Finding	Positive	**True Positive** (Power) $1-\beta$	False Positive Type I Error α
	Negative α	False Negative Type II Error β	**True Negative**

A word on Type I and Type II errors. I remember spending hours on this table in a research methods class, some students did not understand why such a table or concept existed, others were 100% onboard with the concept. You have probably seen this before, but just in case you have not, check out Table 3.6.

Chi-square tests are used to compare two groups of categorical data (data that can be counted or grouped into categories). The Chi-square is noted by the 'X²' symbol and is used to measure the distribution of data and values. **T-tests** are used to answer the question, "Is the difference between two samples different (significant) enough to say that something else could have caused the difference?" **Correlation analyses** is used to describe the strength and linear relationship between two variables. The 'r' value will always be between +1 and -1 where a -1.00 represents a perfect negative linear relationship, and +1.00 represents a perfect positive linear relationship. **Analysis of Variance (ANOVA)** can help evaluators determine if there is a statistically significant difference between three or more groups based on mean scores. ANOVAs are used to determine the mean effect of an intervention or experimental treatment. The main utility of ANOVA is to compare how much one might expect means to spread out if all groups were sampled from the same population, and there were no population differences. Other inferential statistic methods include **Analysis of Covariance (ANCOVA),** regression analyses, factor analysis, multidimensional scaling, cluster analysis, and many others. Multiple regression can be used to explain or predict an outcome. These analyses require a specific computer software and a more advanced understanding of statistics (Kelley, 2018). I would like to add more on regression, but we still have content to cover, and there are **hundreds of textbooks already written on regression,** check out the Resources Section at the end of this chapter for more on regression.

Software programs can help evaluators with the analysis, here are some of my favorites: IBM SPSS (https://www.ibm.com/products/spss-statistics/pricing), STATA (https://www.stata.com/), SAS (https://www.sas.com/en_us/home.html), R (https://www.r-project.org), Excel (https://products.office.com/en-us/excel), and Tableau for data visualization (https://tableau.com) (Kelley, 2018).

Analyzing Qualitative Data

Two years ago, I taught a qualitative analysis workshop to a group of epidemiologists. Some were completely against the concept of using words instead of numbers. Others were completely into the idea that words could be used in evaluation and research in ways that numbers never could. If you find yourself wondering what to do with qualitative data, do not stress. Here are some qualitative analysis strategies: write margin notes, reflect on data, write summary notes, use metaphors, create codes and memos, note patterns and themes, count the frequency of codes (or how often qualitative text appears), note how information is related to outcomes of interests (to build a chain of evidence), and contrast and compare data. I recommend no more than 25 total codes and five to seven themes; evaluators must focus on the relationship of data to outcomes of interest and the overall meaning.

Qualitative data analysis is an entire discipline, it stands alone with experts, evaluators, and advocates specializing in this method of evidence generation and meaning finding. Evaluators often utilize more than 20 different qualitative approaches and strategies. These include ethnography, case study, narrative inquiry, evaluation research, critical inquiry, grounded theory content analysis, arts-based, action research, autoethnography, phenomenology, mixed methods, investigative journalism, historical methods, clinical research, ethnography, life history, testimonio (Creswell & Poth, 2016; Denzin & Lincoln, 2011; Saldana, 2011).

Creswell and Poth describe a spiral when working with qualitative data and the following steps: (1) collect data, (2) manage and organize data, (3) read and memo emergent ideas, (4) describe and classify codes into themes, (5) develop and assess interpretations, (6) represent and visualize findings, and (7) report findings (Creswell & Poth, 2016). Here are some common definitions used in the qualitative analysis milieu. A **code** is a word, phrase, sentence or paragraph that describes a phenomenon and is a meaning unit. **Deductive coding** starts with predefined set of codes from theory, research or interest. **Inductive coding** or open coding starts with nothing, and codes created are generated from data. **Themes** are broad concepts that combine categories from codes to find meaning. A **codebook** includes the name of codes, a description, and an example. **Memos** are short codes, ideas, or phrases that occur.

Here are some general recommendations for analyzing qualitative data.

- Get familiar with the data.
- Identify concepts, ideas, themes, and questions.
- Create codes and definitions for each code before you begin or during the analysis process.
- Assign codes to units of text, images, recordings, or other forms of qualitative data.
- Code data using paper and pen or a computer program like NVivo.
- When possible, two people should code data independently, then come back together to discuss codes, differences, and find agreement in codes developed.
- Summarize the coded data and look for patterns, relationships, frequency of codes, and connect these to your critical evaluation question.
- Reduce codes into themes.
- Share results in a way that is meaningful to the program, community, or evaluation (Kelley, 2018).

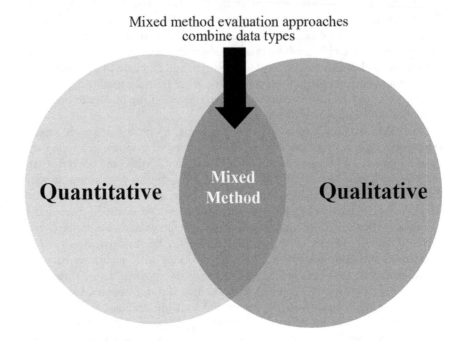

Figure 3.6 Mixed Method Approaches.

Software programs can help with the analysis process, here are some of my favorites: NVivo, QSR International (http://www.qsrinternational.com/nvivo/nvivo-products), QDA Miner and QDA Miner Lite (https://provalisresearch.com/products/qualitative-data-analysis-software/), ATLAS.ti (https://atlasti.com/), MAXQDA (https://www.maxqda.com/). If you want more on qualitative data and analysis approaches (Figure 3.6) used in the evaluation of treatment programs check out Chapters 5 and 6.

Analyzing Mixed Methods Data

You will likely have a mix of quantitative and qualitative data. Quantitative and qualitative analytic procedures described previously may be used when analyzing mixed data.

When you are working with two different kinds of data, determine how data will be transformed and analyzed. One example of data transformation is coding qualitative data and counting the number of times that codes and themes appear in the data (quantification) (Creswell & Poth, 2016; Kelley, 2018). Another example of mixed methods analyses in evaluation is supporting quantitative data with qualitative data. Interviews with survey respondents can help clarify questions in the evaluation, document perspectives and meaning that are not available with quantitative data. Table 3.7 outlines qualitative perspectives from a recent survey

Table 3.7 Example of Codes and Exemplars from Mixed Method Data

Codes	Count	Percentage (%)	Exemplar
Education barriers	43	43	My grades were good but now they are bad. There are lots of barriers I am facing.
Activities	33	33	I am not able to participate in activities and everything has been cancelled.

we conducted with youth involved in an early intervention program. We asked 100 youth how COVID-19 has impacted them. They responded using open-text (typed via online survey). We analyzed these data using NVivo. The code represents the meaning of the text, the count is the number of times the code occurred, and the exemplar is qualitative text from a survey response. A word on weighting. **Weighting** is used to adjust for differences in the sample, for example more women than men. I typically do not weight samples unless it is absolutely necessary, and the sample size is sufficient (>100). Weighting can be avoided if you plan your sampling strategy in advance. Use weighting with caution and consult a statistical textbook or resource at the end of this Chapter for more information.

How you treat qualitative data, and the quantification of data depends on the critical evaluation question, reporting requirements, and how well the data fit.

Step 7. Share Results

Once the evaluation is complete, and you have findings from steps 1–6 it is time to share results. I recommend engaging treatment program staff and stakeholders in the reporting process. Follow this simple five step process for sharing results: 1) engage stakeholders (early and throughout the evaluation), 2) define audience, 3) plan dissemination, 4) know the purpose of the report, and 5) report findings (Kelley, 2018). Evaluators should embrace a public health approach and elevate equity, advocate for policy change, educate people about addiction as a disease and social justice issue, and include marginalized and underrepresented groups in the reporting process (as data collectors, interviewees, reviewers of reports, and recovery advocates). Other uses of evaluation results include social norming, addressing stigma, and promoting access to treatment programs.

Some evaluation reports are used to add knowledge or understanding about a treatment approach or program. Other evaluation reports provide context about what is happening and recommendations for future work. Evaluation reports may also be used in other reports, communications, or policy. Importantly, evaluation reports may establish and reinforce accountability by describing how a program worked and aspects of an intervention that had the greatest effect, along with challenges encountered. **Methods of dissemination** include publishing program and policy briefs, publication in peer-reviewed journals, presentations at conferences, presentation to treatment program staff and partners, reports for funding agencies, press releases, local radio, social media, YouTube, Linked In, health fairs, and via printed program materials like booklets, flyers, posters, and pamphlets. Check out the Resources Section at the end of this chapter for reporting and dissemination resources.

Before we close this chapter let's review evaluation for sustainability and policy change. Why not?

Evaluation for Sustainability and Policy Change

Evaluation findings are powerful, they give a voice to the people and context while influencing policy, social planning, social justice, and transformation (Kelley, 2020). A **policy** is a law, regulation, procedure, action, incentive, or voluntary practices of communities, governments, or other institution. **Policy evaluations** utilize systematic data collection and analysis methods to make decisions about the policy process (Centers for Disease Control, 2019). Policy enactment, adoption, implementation, update, and enforcement are often short-term outcomes highlighted in the program logic model (if the focus is on policy). Program evaluations may target specific policies or identify short and long-term outcomes and impacts related to policy uptake (Kelley, 2018, 2020). **Sustainability** is a method of using a resource so that it is not depleted or permanently changed. Programs, communities, and funding agencies have varied definitions of sustainability (Kelley, 2020). The Substance Abuse and Mental Health Services Administration (SAMHSA) defines prevention program sustainability as, " ... developing prevention systems that promote and support the delivery of effective prevention strategies in order to prevent and reduce substance use, misuse and abuse among whole populations." SAMSHA's sustainability toolkit recommends five steps for evaluation to promote sustainability: (1) document effectiveness of innovation as measured by specific treatment outcomes, (2) document current resources, (3) focus on priority options and opportunities for future funding, (4) assess sustainability innovations and resource options, and (5) institutionalize changes through documentation, dissemination, and leadership (Substance Abuse and Mental Health Services Administration, 2018). Ultimately, sustainability is about maintaining positive outcomes in treatment populations and communities. Treatment programs may have their own definitions of sustainability and policy change.

Renewal Treatment, Inc Sustainability Example

I love examples and I bet you do too. The best way to describe sustainability evaluation is to show one. Here is an example of a sustainability-focused evaluation from Renewal Treatment, Inc. Renewal Treatment, Inc (RTI) is a community based correction organization located in Allegheny County, PA. RTI provides treatment services to adult men and women in the criminal justice system. A recent program evaluation of RTI's efforts reviewed administrative records, client self-report survey and interview data, and court-related data. Evaluators identified four questions: (1) What kind and how much treatment did clients get? (2) Did the program reduce recidivism rates? (3) How are clients doing after the program? And (4) Do clients think that the program helped them?

A program evaluation for a residential drug and alcohol treatment program found that the RTI program reduces recidivism and increases cost-savings. RTI participants were 7% less likely to be re-arrested 12 months after their release compared with individuals in the same county who were not involved in RTI programming. RTI participants were less likely to be arrested after one year compared with individuals who went directly to their homes (rather than community corrections). RTI evaluators also reported a cost-savings of $1,600 per participant in future processing and victimization costs (Williams, 2018).

If you are feeling a bit overwhelmed or perhaps disappointed with the lack of evaluation examples in this chapter, do not fret, Chapter 5 is an entire chapter dedicated to examples of treatment program evaluations.

Wrap Up

We started this chapter by learning about standards and principles for evaluators working in a variety of public health and treatment settings. Know that the field of evaluation is deep, with multiple disciplines, policies, accrediting bodies, and practices guiding the work of evaluators just like you and me. We reviewed a **seven-step process** for treatment program evaluation beginning with the logic modelling process. Logic models are a fun way to outline what you think, hope, or theorize will happen as the result of a program or intervention. Specific examples from a treatment program alternative pain management approach demonstrates how logic models are helpful in outlining desired outcomes. Treatment programs have a variety of activities they implement based on the type of treatment facility they are, and the clients served. Recall in Chapter 1 the Continuum of Care, activities within treatment program settings are guided by the completion requirements. For example, a Level 1.0 treatment facility may provide outpatient services and a minimum of 84 treatment hours completed. Level 1.0 may include recovery or motivational enhancement therapies and strategies delivered in a variety of settings. Developing critical evaluation questions was the third step in the evaluation process, and potentially the most difficult. What must you know and what questions will you ask to gain this knowledge? We cannot ask everything. The next step is selecting an evaluation design (there are many), and then planning to collect data. Collecting data can be a huge undertaking, make sure you have adequate, time, capacity, resources, and data access and use agreements in place. Step 6 is analyzing data and this step depends largely on Steps 1–5. Step 7 is to share evaluation results. Evaluators generally do not have the authority to share treatment program data or results without explicit permission from the treatment program director or person in charge. Evaluators may work closely with treatment programs to create various products that highlight results and target them to key audiences. Dissemination of results should be approved by the IRB first (if the evaluation was reviewed by an IRB). We will discuss this more in Chapters 5–7.

Discussion Questions

1. What are the seven steps to evaluating a treatment program? Which step is most important and why?
2. What is the purpose of a logic model and when should it be developed in the evaluation?
3. What is the difference between a process evaluation, outcome evaluation, and impact evaluation?
4. Describe study designs used in evaluation, their strengths, limitations, and potential uses in a treatment program evaluation.
5. What are some ways that evaluators can advocate for sustainability of positive outcomes within treatment populations and communities?

Resources

Dissemination

Agency for Healthcare Research and Quality Dissemination Planning Tool, https://www.ahrq.gov/patient-safety/resources/advances/vol4/planning.html

Rural Health Information Hub, https://www.ruralhealthinfo.org/toolkits/rural-toolkit/6/dissemination-methods

Stephanie Evergreen's 1–3–25 Reporting Model, https://stephanieevergreen.com/the-1–3–25-reporting-model/

Cost Effectiveness

World Health Organization Guide to Cost-Effectiveness Analysis, https://www.who.int/choice/publications/p_2003_generalised_cea.pdf

Methods, Power and Sample Size

Addiction Research Methods, Sampling Strategies for Addiction Research, https://onlinelibrary-wiley-com.libproxy.uncg.edu/doi/10.1002/9781444318852.ch3

American Psychological Association Criteria for Evaluation Treatment Guidelines, https://www.apa.org/practice/guidelines/evaluating

Regression Sample Sizes, Gordon Brooks, American Education Research Association, https://files.eric.ed.gov/fulltext/ED412247.pdf

Robert Wood Johnson Foundation Qualitative Research Guidelines Project, http://www.qualres.org/HomeLinc-3684.html

Poverty Action Lab Rules of Thumb for Sample Size, https://www.povertyactionlab.org/sites/default/files/research-resources/2018.03.21-Rules-of-Thumb-for-Sample-Size-and-Power_0.pdf

Tufts-Center for the Evaluation of Value and Risk in Health (CEVR), https://cevr.tuftsmedicalcenter.org/

UCLA Institute for Digital Research and Education Statistical Consulting (G*Power), https://stats.idre.ucla.edu/other/gpower/

References

Althubaiti, A. (2016). *Information bias in health research: Definition, pitfalls, and adjustment methods, 9*, 211–217. 10.2147/JMDH.S104807

American Psychological Association (2002). Criteria for Evaluating Treatment Guidelines. American Psychologist. https://www.apa.org/pubs/journals/features/evaluating.pdf

American Evaluation Association. (n.d.). *What is evaluation?* Retrieved September 3, 2021, from https://www.eval.org/Portals/0/What%20is%20evaluation%20Document.pdf

American Evaluation Association (2018). *Guiding principles for evaluators.* https://www.eval.org/About/Guiding-Principles

Centers for Disease Control (2019). *Policy evaluation for policy and strategy CDC.* (2019, June 18). https://www.cdc.gov/policy/analysis/process/evaluation.html

Creswell, J. W., & Poth, C. N. (2016). *Qualitative inquiry and research design: Choosing among five approaches.* SAGE Publications.

Denzin, N. K., & Lincoln, Y. S. (Eds.). (2011). *The SAGE handbook of qualitative research* (Fourth edition). SAGE Publications, Inc.

Department of Health and Human Services (1999). Substance Abuse Prevention Dollars and Cents: A cost-benefit analysis. SAMHSA. https://www.samhsa.gov/sites/default/files/cost-benefits-prevention.pdf

Economic Cost of Substance Abuse in the United States, 2016. (n.d.). *Recovery centers of America.* Retrieved September 8, 2021, from https://recoverycentersofamerica.com/economic-cost-substance-abuse/

Fairley, M., Humphreys, K., Joyce, V. R., Bounthavong, M., Trafton, J., Combs, A., Oliva, E. M., Goldhaber-Fiebert, J. D., Asch, S. M., Brandeau, M. L., & Owens, D. K. (2021). Cost-effectiveness of treatments for opioid use disorder. *JAMA Psychiatry, 78*(7), 767–777. 10.1001/jamapsychiatry.2021.0247

Faul, F., Erdfelder, E., Lang, A.-G., & Buchner, A. (2007). G*Power 3: A flexible statistical power analysis program for the social, behavioral, and biomedical sciences. *Behavior Research Methods, 39*(2), 175–191. 10.3758/BF03193146

Green, L. L., Fullilove, M. T., & Fullilove, R. E. (1998). Stories of spiritual awakening. *Journal of Substance Abuse Treatment, 15*(4), 325–331. 10.1016/S0740-5472(97)00211-0

Greene, J. (2005). In *Encyclopaedia of evaluation* (pp. 397–398). Sage.

JAP-L. (2018). *Six rules of thumb for determining sample size and statistical power.* Jamell Poverty Action Lab. https://www.povertyactionlab.org/sites/default/files/research-resources/2018.03.21-Rules-of-Thumb-for-Sample-Size-and-Power_0.pdf

Jones, S. R. (2003). An introduction to power and sample size estimation. *Emergency Medicine Journal, 20*(5), 453–458. 10.1136/emj.20.5.453

Kakinami, L., & Conner, K. R. (2010). Sampling strategies for addiction research. In *Addiction research methods* (pp. 27–42). John Wiley & Sons, Ltd. 10.1002/9781444318852.ch3

Kelley, A. (2018). *Evaluation in rural communities.* Routledge. 10.4324/9780429458224

Kelley, A. (2020). *Public health evaluation and the social determinants of health* (Vol. 1–1 online resource (xi, 178 pages): illustrations, maps.). Routledge, Taylor & Francis Group. https://www.taylorfrancis.com/books/9781003047810

Kelley, A. (2021). *An interview with Sadie Posey: AKA evaluation intern and chemistry major at Montana State University.* https://www.allysonkelleypllc.com/post/an-interview-with-sadie-posey-aka-evaluation-intern-and-chemistry-major-at-montana-state-university

Khandker, S. R., Koolwal, G. B., & Samad, H. A. (2009). Handbook on impact evaluation: quantitative methods and practices. World Bank Publications.

Lincoln, Y. S., & Guba, E. G. (1985). *Naturalistic inquiry*. SAGE.

Lipsey, M., & Hurley, S. (2009). Design sensitivity: Statistical power for applied experimental research. In L. Bickman, & D. Rog, *The SAGE handbook of applied social research methods* (pp. 44–76). SAGE Publications, Inc. 10.4135/9781483348858.n2

McLellan, A. T., McKay, J. R., Forman, R., Cacciola, J., & Kemp, J. (2005). Reconsidering the evaluation of addiction treatment: From retrospective follow-up to concurrent recovery monitoring. *Addiction, 100*(4), 447–458. 10.1111/j.1360-0443.2005.01012.x

Morse, J. M. (2000). Determining sample size. *Qualitative Health Research, 10*(1), 3–5. 10.1177/104973200129118183

Mysiak, K. (2020, August 28). *The relationship between significance, power, sample size & effect size*. Medium. https://towardsdatascience.com/the-relationship-between-significance-power-sample-size-effect-size-899fcf95a76d

NIDA (2020, September 18). Principles of Effective Treatment. Retrieved from https://www.drugabuse.gov/publications/principles-drug-addiction-treatment-research-based--guide-third-edition/principles-effective-treatment on 2022, January 24

Padian, N. S., Holmes, C. B., McCoy, S. I., Lyerla, R., Bouey, P. D., & Goosby, E. P. (2011). Implementation science for the US President's Emergency Plan for AIDS Relief (PEPFAR). *Journal of Acquired Immune Deficiency Syndromes (1999), 56*(3), 199–203. 10.1097/QAI.0b013e31820bb448

Palinkas, L. A. (2014). Qualitative methods in mental health services research. *Journal of Clinical Child and Adolescent Psychology: The Official Journal for the Society of Clinical Child and Adolescent Psychology, American Psychological Association, Division 53, 43*(6), 851–861. 10.1080/15374416.2014.910791

Pannucci, C. J., & Wilkins, E. G. (2010). Identifying and avoiding bias in research. *Plastic and Reconstructive Surgery, 126*(2), 619–625. 10.1097/PRS.0b013e3181de24bc

Proctor, E., Silmere, H., Raghavan, R., Hovmand, P., Aarons, G., Bunger, A., Griffey, R., & Hensley, M. (2011). Outcomes for implementation research: Conceptual distinctions, measurement challenges, and research agenda. *Administration and Policy in Mental Health, 38*(2), 65–76. 10.1007/s10488-010-0319-7

Rushing, S. C., Kelley, A., Bull, S., Stephens, D., Wrobel, J., Silvasstar, J., Peterson, R., Begay, C., Dog, T. G., McCray, C., Brown, D. L., Thomas, M., Caughlan, C., Singer, M., Smith, P., & Sumbundu, K. (2021). Efficacy of an mHealth intervention (BRAVE) to promote mental wellness for American Indian and Alaska native teenagers and young adults: Randomized controlled trial. *JMIR Mental Health, 8*(9), e26158. 10.2196/26158

Rural Health Information Hub. (n.d.). *Evaluation Measures—RHIhub Substance Use Disorder Toolkit*. (n.d.). Retrieved September 8, 2021, from https://www.ruralhealthinfo.org/toolkits/substance-abuse/5/evaluation-measures

Saldana, J. (2011). *Fundamentals of qualitative research* (P. Leavy, Ed.; 1st edition). Oxford University Press.

Serdar, C. C., Cihan, M., Yücel, D., & Serdar, M. A. (2021). Sample size, power and effect size revisited: Simplified and practical approaches in pre-clinical, clinical and laboratory studies. *Biochemia Medica, 31*(1), 010502. 10.11613/BM.2021.010502

Setia, M. S. (2016). Methodology series module 5: Sampling strategies. *Indian Journal of Dermatology, 61*(5), 505–509. 10.4103/0019-5154.190118

Substance Abuse and Mental Health Services Administration (n.d.) Substance abuse prevention dollars and cents. Retrieved September 8, 2021, from https://www.samhsa.gov/sites/default/files/cost-benefits-prevention.pdf

Substance Abuse and Mental Health Services Administration (n.d.). Strategic prevention framework. Retrieved September 10, 2021, from https://www.samhsa.gov/sites/default/files/20190620-samhsa-strategic-prevention-framework-guide.pdf

Substance Abuse and Mental Health Services Administration. (2018). *Sustainability-Toolkit-508*. 78. https://ncsacw.samhsa.gov/files/sustainability-toolkit-508.pdf

Telfair, J., Kelley, A., & Dave, G. (2022). *Chapter 19 program monitoring and evaluation. In Kotch's maternal and child health* (R. S. Kirby & S. Verbiest, Eds.; 4th edition). Jones & Bartlett Learning.

Watson, P. (2019). How to screen for ACEs in an efficient, sensitive, and effective manner. *Paediatrics & Child Health*, 24(1), 37–38. 10.1093/pch/pxy146

Williams, J. (2018, May 2). Program evaluation for a residential drug and alcohol program. *Institute for Research, Education, and Training in Addictions*. https://ireta.org/case_studies/program-evaluation-for-a-residential-drug-and-alcohol-program/

Wrobel, J., Silvasstar, J., Peterson, R., Sumbundu, K., Kelley, A., Stephens, D., Craig Rushing, S., & Bull, S. (2021). Text messaging intervention for mental wellness in American Indian and Alaska Native teens and young adults (BRAVE Study): Analysis of user engagement patterns. *JMIR Formative Research*. 2021 Nov 22. doi: . [Epub ahead of print]10.2196/32138

4 The System that Supports Recovery

CONTENTS

DOI: 10.4324/9781003290728-4

Learning Objectives

After reading this chapter, you should be able to:

- Summarize recovery principles and how they are operationalized within recovery contexts.
- List the four models of social support used in recovery systems and settings.
- Discuss Recovery Oriented Systems of Care, approaches, barriers, and solutions.
- Describe systems that support recovery and evaluation examples from the field.

What does it mean to recover? How do systems support recovery and why does recovery even matter? Recovery is about developing a new way of living in the world (Anthony, 1993). Recovery has been defined as "a deeply personal, unique process of change … a way of living a satisfying, hopeful and contributing life even with limitations caused by illness [and] a process involving the development of new meaning or purpose in one's life" ([3] p. 527).

September is recovery month. Throughout the world recovery advocates, clinicians, programs, funders, evaluators, researchers, families, and individuals celebrate recovery.

Recovery month is about celebrating these four messages…

1. Behavioral health is essential to health
2. Prevention works
3. Treatment is effective
4. People recover

If you are evaluating a MHSU program, it is likely that your work involves some aspect of recovery. From an individual perspective, it is possible that you yourself, are in recovery. Recovery is about reclaiming and regaining what has been lost (within individuals and programs). Systems and evaluators support individuals and MHSU programs as they make this reclaiming possible.

Here are some examples of how an MHSU evaluation team promotes recovery through evaluation (Kelley, 2021).

- Evaluators recognize that we are all in recovery. Every organization, individual, community, program, and evaluation has recovered from something. This acknowledgement is the common ground that connects evaluators to people, places, and systems.
- Evaluators work with funding agencies, state and local governments, tribes, recovery centers, recovery coaches, clinicians, individuals in recovery, families, youth, policy makers, and communities that support recovery.

- Evaluators document what has been lost so that MHSU programs can fill gaps, create policies, and do better. Evaluators dive deep into MHSU programs and services to find out how the recovery and regaining process is happening and evidence to support this knowing.
- Evaluators seek to find out what supports recovery in MHSU programs. This seeking tells evaluators about what is working, the transforming of individuals, families, communities, and systems.
- Evaluators explore and test what works, through various forms of data collection, analysis, and reporting. This furthers understanding about about loss and brokenness so that wholeness is possible.
- Evaluators elevate the voice of individuals and programs in recovery, making evaluation a platform for public discourse, truth-seeking, story-telling, and courage. This happens in the dissemination of evaluation findings, through podcasts, books, reports, artwork, and more.

Recovery Capital

Systems that support recovery build recovery capital. Recovery capital is the amount of resources that people need to initiate or sustain recovery from substance misuse. Authors describe four types of recovery capital (Granfield & Cloud, 2001; M. White, 2008). **Personal recovery capital** includes both physical and human capital. **Physical recovery capital** is everything people need physically to maintain health (food, shelter, transportation, healthcare, and financial resources). **Human recovery capital** includes abilities, skills, education, self-efficacy, self-regulation abilities, healthy coping, interpersonal skills, and being able to navigate difficult situations. **Family and social recovery capital** are resources and relationships with family and friends, others in recovery, and access to recovery activities and events. **Community recovery capital** may include attitudes, norms, ideas, policies, beliefs, and resources about recovery. These might include activity, advocacy, recovery community organizations, institutional support from schools and faith-based organizations. **Cultural recovery capital** includes what people believe and have faith in (e.g., Christianity). Recovery programs are systems that support recovery and recovery capital.

Public Health Takeaway- Recovery capital is developed within individuals, families, and communities. A public health approach advocates for understanding what causes MHSUD and addressing the risk and protective factors that are associated with resilience, recovery, and health and wellness (step 2).

Recovery Programs

There are many systems that support recovery. In this chapter we focus on three types of recovery programs--there are many (National Institute on Drug Abuse, 2017). (Figure 4.1)

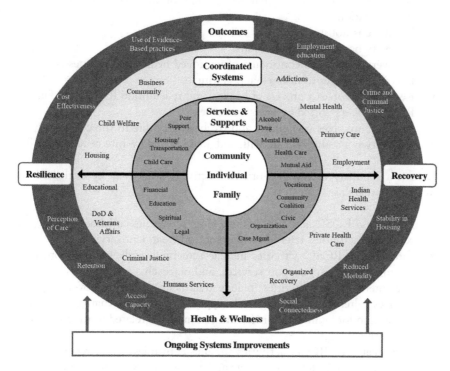

Figure 4.1 Recovery Oriented Systems of Care (ROSC).

- Recovery-oriented systems of care (ROSC)
- Recovery support services
- Social and recreational recovery infrastructures and social media

Evaluators are part of systems at MHSU programs that support recovery, and there are multiple smaller systems that support recovery along the way. SAMHSA's recovery-oriented systems of care (ROSC) are widely used throughout the United States (SAMHSA, 2020).

SAMHSA describes ROSC as, "a coordinated network of community-based services and supports that is person-centered and builds on the strengths and resiliencies of individuals, families, and communities to achieve abstinence and improved health, wellness, and quality of life for those with or at risk of alcohol and drug problems" (SAMHSA, 2010, p. 2). William White and colleagues write about the benefits of state-led ROSC and guiding principles of recovery, and of ROSC approaches. Guiding Principles of Recovery are outlined below.

- There are many pathways to recovery.
- Recovery is self-directed and empowering.

- Recovery involves a personal recognition of the need for change and transformation.
- Recovery is holistic.
- Recovery has cultural dimensions.
- Recovery exists on a continuum of improved health and wellness.
- Recovery emerges from hope and gratitude.
- Recovery involves a process of healing and redefinition for self and family.
- Recovery is supported by peers and allies.
- Recovery involves (re)joining and (re)building a life in the community.
- Recovery is a reality. It can, will, and does happen (White & Kurtz, 2008).

Here is a summary of recovery-oriented activities that may be evaluated by treatment programs.

- Prevention ROSC activities include early screening, collaboration, stigma reduction activities, referral to intervention treatment services.
- Intervention ROSC activities include screening, early intervention, pre-treatment, recovery support services, and outreach.
- Treatment ROSC activities include treatment services, recovery support services, alternative healing and support services, alternative therapies, prevention for families, abilities, and communities related to the individual in treatment.
- Post-treatment ROSC activities include continuing care, recovery support, check-ups, self-monitoring, and general relapse prevention efforts (SAMHSA, 2010).

Within each ROSC the mission, values, goals, system elements, and core functions lead to desired recovery-related outcomes (SAMHSA, 2010). The **mission of a ROSC** may be to improve health, wellness, recovery and healing for individuals, families, communities, and nations who are placed at risk of MHSU problems, while promoting healthy, safe, and vibrant communities. **Values** are developed within an ROSC, some recovery values include person-centered, strength-based, family engaged, community-supported, and healing focused. Goals also vary by MHSU programs within an ROSC but may include to prevent SUD, to intervene early, to support recovery, or to improve outcomes. **System elements** are also ROSC context dependent, but may include integrated, community-based, outcomes drive, collaborative, peer, and community driven, and flexible. Core functions within an ROSC vary but could include education, dissemination, advocacy, implementation of policy and practice changes, service delivery, service coordination, quality improvement, and use of a public health approach to recovery. Ultimately ROSC outcomes focus on improvements to access, quality, and effectiveness. These outcomes are closely tied to systems elements and core functions.

Systems that support recovery are at every level from prevention, intervention, treatment, and post-treatment. These systems are located in churches, schools, groups, organizations, agencies, treatment facilities, county health departments, and many others.

Recovery Support Services

When you think about recovery support services, what comes to mind? For some people it is 12-step groups, AA and NA programs, recovery coaching, recovery housing, recovery management, recovery community centers, and recovery-based education. The common thread linking all of these services is that they support individuals in recovery using a variety of methods. One well-known federally funded program is the **Recovery Community Support Program (RCSP).** RCSP stresses **four models of social support including informational, instrumental, emotional, and affiliation**. Evaluators may work with treatment centers to explore each of these models of support in more detail, for example **informational support** may include training and education and evaluators may develop instruments that assess knowledge, information, and skills gained by participants after completing a training program. **Instrumental support** may be assessed by counting the frequency of services provided including transportation, assistance completing job application forms, food assistance, childcare, or transportation. Evaluators may capture impacts of **emotional support** by assessing mentoring, coaching, or recovery support services offered. **Affiliational support** is the last model of support and evaluators may assess affiliational support by examining how well individuals feel connected to their social groups or communities.

Recovery Coaches and Peer Recovery Support Specialists (PRSS)

Systems that support recovery often include Peer Recovery Support Specialists (PRSS). These peer-led positions are sometimes called recovery coaches, patient navigators, peer recovery specialist, recovery coach, or peer navigator. Regardless of title, these individuals have the lived experience of recovery and have completed at least one 40-hour certification PRSS course. States have different requirements for PRSS but the goals of PRSS are the same, to empower individuals, to decrease substance use, improve quality of life, promote self-esteem and sense of purpose. PRSS services include emotional, informational, instrumental, and affiliational (Reif et al., 2014). PRSS collaborate with individuals in recovery to support them as they seek education and training programs, employment, sober housing, and navigate the criminal justice system. PRSS may be offered to individuals at any point in their recovery process (Eddie et al., 2019). Eddie and colleagues conducted a systematic review of PRSS and found that PRSS improved relationships with treatment providers, increased social supports, increased treatment retention, and improved satisfaction with treatment (Eddie et al., 2019). More research is needed to fully understand the impacts of PRSS on recovery since most research on PRSS is limited to clinical SUD populations.

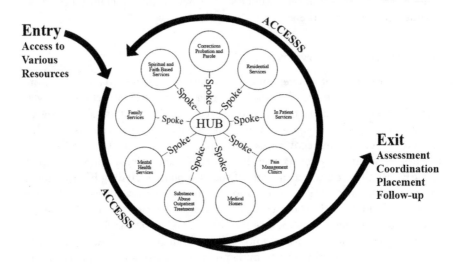

Figure 4.2 Hub and Spoke Model.

The **Hub and Spoke model** is an example of a recovery system and various recovery supports available within a system. This model connects providers around a central hub that provides various MHSU supports for individuals seeking services. This model works because it assumes that individuals seeking services will enter the system at various locations, not just one. Designers of this tested model use it to extend spokes, collaborate with providers, subcontract with other locations, and ensure that every individual receives the care that they need. (Figure 4.2)

Vermont has one of the most well-known Hub-and-Spoke models of care for opioid use disorder. In the last 5 years, Vermont's Hub-and-Spoke model has been implemented and adopted by providers and patients (Brooklyn and Sigmon, 2017). Researchers report that because of the model, the state's treatment capacity for OUD increased, where the state of Vermont has the highest capacity for treatment in the United States (Brooklyn and Sigmon, 2017). This model also increased the number of physicians waivered to prescribe buprenorphine, and increased patient access to medication assisted treatment (Brooklyn and Sigmon, 2017).

12-Steps and Alcoholics Anonymous (AA) and Narcotics Anonymous (NA)

Founded in 1939, AA is the largest alcohol and drug related 12-step programs in the world (Sussman, 2010). AA is a self-governing, nonprofit organization whose only requirement for membership is a desire to stop drinking (Galanter, 2007). AA programs utilize approaches informed by cognitive behavioral therapy (CBT) and motivational treatment (MT), but not in a clinical setting (see Chapter 2). Developed following principles of the Oxford Group, a religious organization that wanted to replicate Christianity but without doctrine, the 12-step programs today welcome all people and faiths, while promoting the concept of a higher power and spiritual experiences. As one of the most widely known and used recovery support programs, AA is located in 150 countries and includes more than 2 million members (White & Kurtz, 2008).

The 12-steps of AA include the following:

1. We admitted we were powerless over alcohol—that our lives had become unmanageable.
2. Came to believe that a Power greater than ourselves could restore us to sanity.
3. Made a decision to turn our will and our lives over to the care of God as we understood Him.
4. Made a searching and fearless moral inventory of ourselves.
5. Admitted to God, to us, and to another human being the exact nature of our wrongs.
6. Were entirely ready to have God remove all these defects of character.
7. Humbly asked Him to remove our shortcomings.
8. Made a list of all persons we had harmed and became willing to make amends to them all.
9. Made direct amends to such people wherever possible, except when to do so would injure them or others.
10. Continued to take personal inventory and when we were wrong promptly admitted it.
11. Sought through prayer and meditation to improve our conscious contact with God as we understood Him, praying only for knowledge of His will for us and the power to carry that out.
12. Having had a spiritual awakening as the result of these steps, we tried to carry this message to alcoholics, and to practice these principles in all our affairs (Alcoholics Anonymous, n.d. p. 1).

Since AA's inception in 1939, several recovery programs have replicated AA such as Narcotics Anonymous (NA), Self-Management and Recovery Training (SMART), Women for Sobriety, Rational Recovery, Secular Organization for Sobriety, and LifeRing Secular Recovery (Bradshaw, 2019).

Medicine Wheel/White Bison

The Medicine Wheel is used throughout the world and in American Indian and Alaska Native communities in the United States to demonstrate the importance of mental, spiritual, emotional, and physical wellbeing as they relate to recovery. White Bison is a 12-step recovery program that utilizes the Medicine Wheel and the 12-steps in communities throughout the US. The program focuses on Native

Americans who are completing treatment, returning to the community from incarceration, or who have been working on their recovery journey and wish to provide support to others experiencing similar situations. The Medicine Wheel and 12-step program is designed in a series of modules that enable people to meet their individual needs. For example, steps 1 through 3 focus on Finding the Creator; steps 4–6 focus on Finding Yourself; steps 7–9 focus on Finding Your Relationship with others; steps 10–12 focus on Finding the Wisdom of the Elders (Kemppainen et al., 2008). White Bison advocates for **the Four Laws of Change** in their recovery model, including 1) change comes from within, 2) for development to occur, it must be preceded by a vision, 3) a great learning must occur, and 4) you must create a healing forest. Recovery programs may use a video, presentation, or small group that explains Medicine Wheel teachings and how they can be applied to a participant's own life. The Medicine Wheel strengthens social and emotional bonds among participants and fosters emotional, mental, physical, and spiritual growth (Coyhis & Simonelli, 2005). A key difference between the Medicine Wheel program and a 12-step program is the incorporation of Native values and spirituality. For example, each step includes a value that participants embrace, such as honesty, hope, faith, courage, integrity, humility, and service.

12 Step Steps for Men (Coyhis & Simonelli, 2005)

- Finding the Creator - Steps 1, 2, 3
- Finding Yourself - Steps 4, 5, 6
- Finding Your Relationship With Others - Steps 7, 8, 9
- Finding the Wisdom of Elders - Steps 10, 11, 12

White Bison's Wellbriety and Firestarter Curriculum

White Bison implemented a peer-designed and peer-delivered curriculum from 1998 to 2008 based on Native American traditional values and the Four Laws of Change for Wellbriety. Peer leaders, also called Firestarter's, are trained to mobilize and implement change in their communities (Moore & Coyhis, 2010). Working to empower local communities to provide peer support, recovery support services, prevention, address stigmatization, and increase local resources, the Wellbriety program model reported positive outcomes from peer service system implementation. Briefly, 300 communities participated in Hoop Journeys, where volunteers participated in 3-day Firestarter trainings. Before each training participants completed a survey with standardized indicators about health and social behaviors. This survey was administered again to the same people 6 months after the Firestarter training. Findings from baseline to post-training show that Firestarter's helped create peer led community service networks, including reentry programs for individuals in prison or treatment. The training also created a pool of volunteers that supported individuals through faith, school, and social service programs. Outcome indicators demonstrate increases in participation in nonfaith/religious self-help groups and family and friends recovery support. Prosocial indicators by a crime-free lifestyle increased 3.2%, employment and or school enrollment increased 6.4%, and negative substance related personal social consequences improved 3.3% (Moore & Coyhis, 2010).

Healing Forest Concept

White Bison and other social theorists advocate for the concept of a healing forest. The Healing Forest model is based on the idea that if one tree in a forest is sick and removed, and brought back to health, then returned to a sick forest, the tree will become sick again. Healing communities require everyone's participation in the healing process. Moore and Coyhis advocate that this is the only way systemic change will occur. The roots of the forest must address anger, guilt, shame, and fear. The new roots must be based in culture and spirituality (Moore & Coyhis, 2010). The soil and conditions surrounding the forest must be healthy, vibrant, nutrient dense, feeding the roots so that every tree thrives.

Recovery Homes and Housing

Recovery homes (RHs) support individuals in recovery and are classified using four levels. Level 1 RHs are self-run without support from professionals. Level 2 RHs have a peer or professional on site to support recovery-related activities and services. Level 3 RHs include professionals in the home, clinical services, and service coordination. Level 4 RHs are generally licensed with clinical services, state-funded services, court-mandated living, and often times coordinate services with larger instructions (Jason et al., 2021). Housing programs support individuals in recovery by providing alcohol and drug free living environments. One of the most popular recovery housing program approaches is Oxford House (Oxford House, 2021). Oxford Houses are recovery homes for individuals with substance abuse histories and there are more than 1200 of them in the United States (Jason et al., 2006). The Oxford House Model is based on the following guidelines:

1. May be democratically self-run
2. Membership is responsible for all expenses
3. Individuals in recovery may live in the house as long as they do not drink alcohol, use drugs, and pay equal expenses
4. If anyone uses substances they are expelled
5. Average stay is about a year, but some people stay up to 3 years
6. Houses are men-only or women-only houses
7. Applications to live in houses are received by existing members of the house
8. Houses have six to ten members
9. No limits placed on sobriety, some individuals are sober for 5 days, others 30 or more (Jason et al., 2006).

Evaluation of the Oxford House model shows that substance use and criminal activity decreased, and employment improved for individuals living in an Oxford House compared with individuals assigned to "usual care" (Jason et al., 2006). An essential part of the Oxford House model is the recovery support network that is available to residents. Recovery support networks provide mentoring, support for abstinence related goals, and self-improvement, all of which support long-term recovery.

A longitudinal evaluation of Level 2 RHs found that when residents are engaged in 12-step groups they are more likely to maintain long-term recovery (Borkman et al., 1998). Research also suggests that individuals who live in RHs with clinical support and stay longer have better outcomes than individuals who do not have clinical support or shorter stays (Polcin et al., 2010). Many RHs utilize 12-step programs like the Medicine Wheel and White Bison to support American Indian/Alaska Native populations and others in recovery.

Education at High Schools and Colleges

Education-based recovery systems help individuals achieve their educational and career goals, while in recovery (Recovery Research Institute, n.d.). At the university level, **Collegiate Recovery Programs (CRPs)** connect individuals with recovery-related supports such as sober housing, AA groups, sober events, counseling, and various student groups that support recovery. There are more than 138 active CRPs in the US, led by peers in recovery, and based in a 12-step abstinence framework. National research on CRPs is somewhat limited, but one study at Texas Tech University's CRP found that relapse rates were just 4% to 8% among CRP participants and 70% of CRP participants graduated, which was more than the general student population graduation rate (Jason et al., 2021). **Recovery High Schools (RHSs)** support students in recovery from SUD and co-occurring disorders by providing them with a therapeutic environment that supports retention and academic performance. According to the Association of Recovery Schools there are 45 recovery high schools in the United States and eight of these are located in Texas (Association of Recovery Schools, 2021). A recent study of 194 adolescents enrolled at RHSs in Minnesota, Wisconsin, and Texas found that students in RHSs were less likely to use alcohol, marijuana, and other drugs at 6-month follow-up compared with non-RHS students. Students enrolled in RHSs were also more likely to attend school than non-RHS students (Finch et al., 2018).

Families as Recovery Support Systems

Families play an essential role in the recovery process and are systems within themselves. Research suggests that when families participate in recovery, individuals are more likely to adhere to treatment regimens and have positive recovery outcomes compared with individuals without family support (Kennedy & Horton, 2011). Researchers conducted a multimethod study of behavioral health reform in New Mexico and interviewed 14 behavioral health agencies to explore family systems that support recovery. Types of assistance offered by family members to individuals include being there, emotional or moral aid, encouraging social activity, encouraging treatment, feedback, financial, general, going to appointments, childcare, housing, listening, making appointments, reading, writing, match, forms, socializing, self-care, transportation, understanding, and other types of assistance (Kennedy & Horton, 2011). Families as systems play an essential role to individuals as they move back into their communities and families and create systems of support that promote recovery.

Social and Recreational Recovery Infrastructures and Social Media

Social media may help or hinder recovery. The current pandemic drastically impacted the recovery community and in-person programs that support recovery. Individuals in recovery report stress, isolation, limited access to health care, difficulty accessing treatment, and lack of structure as key factors that threaten their recovery (McDonnell et al., 2021). During the pandemic, many treatment programs switched to online groups, telehealth sessions, and one-on-one chats as opposed to in-person sessions. Social media and virtual sessions were instrumental in connecting people to wellness resources.

Digital Recovery Support Services (D-RSS)

D-RSS tools are increasingly being used to support individuals through telehealth platforms, recovery apps, and remote monitoring (wearable devices). Examples of D-RSS include websites, digital recovery forums, social networking sites based in recovery, smartphone applications, and text messaging programs. Although researchers do not have convincing evidence that D-RSS promotes recovery-related outcomes, they are widely used. A recent study by Ashford and colleagues reports that at least 11% of US adults who are in recovery from a SUD have used at least one D-RSS tool (Ashford et al., 2020). A benefit of D-RSS is they eliminate barriers that many experience when seeking recovery such as confidentiality, anonymity, scheduling conflicts, childcare, work schedules, transportation, and others. Importantly, D-RSS make recovery accessible. A systematic review of D-RSS users found that low income individuals were more likely to use D-RSS than a national recovery study sample (Bergman et al., 2018).

Social Media and Networks

Social networks (from social media) and social capital are predictors of health and well-being. Social factors are associated with alcohol and drug abuse (both recovery and relapse). Mowbray and colleagues explored social ties and networks in a national sample of adults with varying use and social networking characteristics (2014). Individuals without an AUD history had the largest social networks. Conversely, individuals with AUD reported the smallest social networks. Authors call for social network interventions focused on reducing alcohol use within social network settings (Mowbray et al., 2014; Owens & McCrady, 2014). Owens and colleagues reviewed social environments and their impact on alcohol or drug relapse in persons recently released from jail (2014). They found that adult males' social networks change after spending time in jail and social networks predict an individual's future substance use. Researchers indicate that when participants did not change their social network 1 month after being released from jail, they were more likely to continue their pattern of substance use (Owens & McCrady, 2014). Most treatment programs agree that people in early recovery should be careful about engaging with social media and what they post on various social media platforms (Smith, 2019). When individuals post about their recovery online, they may be subject to stigmatization, judgement, and employer reviews of online presence and activities. Recovery.org encourages people to post on social media in a closed group with members that individuals know (Smith, 2019). Some recommend waiting up to a year to publicly share recovery stories with others. Future work could develop specific interventions that target the release date. Doing so may reduce criminal activity, future substance use, and the likelihood of returning back to jail. All result in significant cost savings and improvement to overall public health.

Individual and Organizational Recovery Measures

One approach for measuring recovery capital is the **Assessment of Recovery Capital (ARC) instrument.** ARC assesses 10 recovery capital domains including the following, 1) substance use and sobriety (e.g., "I am currently completely sober), 2) global health (e.g., I am able to concentrate when I need to)., 3) global physical health (e.g., I cope well with everyday tasks), 4) citizenship and community involvement (e.g., I am proud of the community I live in and feel part of it-sense of belonging), 5) social support (e.g., I am happy with my personal life), 6) meaningful activities (e.g., I am actively involved in leisure and sport activities), 7) housing and safety (e.g., I am proud of my home), 8) risk taking (e.g., I am free from worries about money), 9) coping and life functioning (e.g., I am happy dealing with a range of professional people), 10) recovery experience (e.g., I am making good progress on my recovery journey) (Groshkova et al., 2013).

Previous researchers have explored indicators of recovery utilizing client focus groups and Delphi group techniques (Neale et al., 2016). Neale and colleagues published **76 indicators of recovery** (2016). Indicators are based on the categories of substance use, treatment/support, psychological health, physical health, use of time, education/training/employment, income, housing, relationships, social functioning, offending/anti-social behaviour, well-being, identity/self-awareness, goals and aspirations. Table 4.1 is an example of how indicators of recovery could be operationalized in a treatment program evaluation.

Stevens and colleagues conducted a review of individual and organizational recovery measures that met the following inclusion criteria: holistic recovery,

Table 4.1 Example Recovery Measures

Drinking and Drug use
 1. I have drunk too much
 2. I have used street drugs
 3. I have abused medication prescribed to me by a doctor
 4. I have experienced cravings
Mental Health
 5. I have been looking after my mental health
 6. I have coped with problems without turning to drugs or alcohol
 7. I have felt emotionally stable and secure
 8. I have felt that I am a worthwhile person
Physical Health
 9. I have been looking after my physical health
 10. I have managed pains and ill-health without misusing drugs or alcohol
 11. I have been taking care of my appearance
 12. I have been eating a good diet
 13. I have slept well
Relationships
 14. I have been getting on well with people
 15. I have had enough company and spent enough time with other people
 16. I have felt supported by people around me
Material Resources
 17. I have had stable housing
 18. I have had a regular income (from benefits, work, or other legal sources)
 19. I have been managing my money well
Daily Activities
 20. I have had a good daily routine
 21. I have been going to my appointments
 22. I have been spending my free time on hobbies and interests that do not involve drinking or drug use
 23. I have been in education, training or work (paid or voluntary)
Outlook on Life
 24. I have felt happy with my overall quality of life
 25. I have felt positive
 26. I have had realistic hopes and goals for myself
Rights and Responsibilities
 27. I have been treated with respect and consideration by people around me
 28. I have treated others with respect and consideration
 29. I have been honest and law-abiding
 30. I have tried to help and support other people

(Neale et al., 2016).

person-centered, evidence, measures change, and accessible (2018). Nine organizational measures and 11 individual measures met their inclusion criteria. They call for use of both individual and organizational measures within a ROSC and advocate for these four organizational measures and three individual measures (note they did not include ARC, but that is okay). **Organizational Measures.** Recovery Self-Assessment (RSA), Recovery Oriented Services Assessment (ROSA), Recovery Oriented Systems Indicator (ROSI), Recovery

Promoting Relationships Scale (RPRS). **Individual Measures**. Recovery Assessment Scale, Maryland Assessment of Recovery, and the Patient Activation Measure (PAM-MH) (Stevens et al., 2018). Check out the Resources section at the end of this Chapter for more information about these recovery measures, authors, psychometrics, and use.

Global Approaches for Systems that Support Recovery

So far, we have reviewed systems that support recovery based on what is happening in the United States. I apologize if this feels Americentric. While the United States writes a ton about systems that support recovery, the systems are lacking. The International Initiative for Mental Health Leadership (IIMHL) led a study to explore ROSC in ten countries throughout the world. IIMHL reviewed the current status of ROSC and measures that would support quality improvement and accountability among countries and nations (Pincus et al., 2016). Here is what they found.

Australia prioritizes recovery, policies, and service standards. Their work includes a framework for recovery-oriented practices including culture and hope, person first, personal recovery, organizational commitment, and social inclusion/determinants. Australia's ROSC appears to be focused on mental health rather than the integration of MHSU. Similarly, the **Mental Health Commission of Canada** is developing recovery guidelines to move toward a recovery-oreinted system for mental health. Canada's framework calls for aligning concepts of recovery, practice shifts, and systems transformation. **England** has been leading a recovery-focused approach since 2001 and their latest effort, No Health Without Mental Health Dashboard, supports several recovery-oriented measures like employment, housing, quality of life, confidence, and other factors. **Germany** developed evidence-based guidelines for the diagnosis and treatment decisions made by mental health providers and service users. **Ireland** called for a recovery-focused perspective in 2006 with the Health Research Board leading recovery-focused efforts. Since 2006, Ireland has made considerable progress toward developing a ROSC, even though the focus is primarily on mental health opposed to SU or MHSU. Advancing Recovery Ireland is one recovery-led initiative that calls for improvements in service level structures, systems, and practices so that recovery support is maximized for all. In the **Netherlands**, recovery-oriented systems are emerging within their mental health systems. They developed a national action plan called Crossing the Bridge for individuals with severe mental illness. This action plan calls for recovery, empowerment, community integration, and combating stigma. **New Zealand** developed a Blueprint strategy paper in 1998 and an updated strategy paper in 2012. New Zealand's Blueprint focuses on elevating mental health and addiction issues. They developed two recovery questions for addiction services that could be replicated in other countries and ROSCs. These questions are: 1) Overall how close are you to where you want to be in your recovery?" (select a number between 1 and 10), and 2) How satisfied are you with your progress towards achieving your recovery goals?" (Not at all, slightly, moderately, considerably, extremely) (Fitzgerald et al., 2016). **Norway** established elements of a recovery-oriented practice framework from 1999 to 2008 and more recently created national guidelines that emphasize recovery-oriented practices for MHSU (Pincus et al., 2016).

Barriers Within Systems that Support Recovery

Systems that support recovery are vital in the prevention, treatment, and follow-up of individuals with MHSUD. However, the implementation and evaluation of ROSC can be difficult.

SAMHSA Expert Panel

SAMHSA gathered experts to attend a 2-day meeting on operationalizing recovery oriented systems for MHSU (SAMHSA, 2012). Experts identified several barriers to operationalizing recovery oriented systems including administrative issues related to program evaluation and desired outcomes, workforce development, lack of cross-system collaboration, and the need for community inclusion. **Administrative barriers** identified include leadership, systems change, and the need for engaged stakeholders. **Program evaluation** and targeted outcome barriers call for more **holistic and comprehensive outcomes** like improved quality of life and well-being measures (opposed to abstinence or reductions in symptoms as the primary outcome of interest). Building the workforce through systems necessary, experts call for transformation, capacity building, and training/hiring certified peer recovery support specialists. **Cross system collaboration issues** include differences in approaches, philosophies, definitions, language, policies, and norms related to MHSU systems. Expert panelists recommend remedying these barriers by amending policies at the local, federal, and state levels. Experts suggest financing and incentivizing services and systems, promoting collaboration, and involving the recovery community in developing cross system supports. Community inclusion is the last barrier identified by expert panelists. A ROSC acknowledges not just the recovery community but also the entire community that is connected to the system. Issues related to community inclusion include the inability to gain employment while participating in a program, lack of ties to community supports outside of the recovery oriented system (for example education, economic, social supports, and housing). Solutions that may support community inclusion are addressing stigma, racism, discrimination, promoting cross-systems collaboration, engaging diverse stakeholder groups, and normalizing treatment and recovery.

Challenges and Recommendations from Pennsylvania ROSC

White and colleagues discuss challenges they encountered when implementing an ROSC including the following (2008):

- Conflicting priorities that shift focus from acute to chronic models of care
- Limited knowledge of what recovery is and means
- Pervasive stigma and discrimination experienced by individuals with addiction
- Limited use or regard for scientific knowledge or evidence that supports the fact that addiction is a brain disease
- Failure to acknowledge the benefits of ROSC on individuals, families, communities, and nations. Fragmented systems and funding issues
- Staff engagement and retention issues
- Limited societal understanding of the benefits of ROSC (White, 2008)

White and colleagues point to systems change rooted within states, counties, tribes, and federal policies and procedures as a solution. Where policies are in place to support the widespread adoption of ROSC and values that undergird the model. White cautions that in order for true systems change to occur, organizations must shift how services are delivered and what the recovery environment looks like. For example, providing individuals with a full menu of ROSC that meets their recovery and wellness needs. Coordination between recovery agencies, licensing and accrediting bodies, and governmental officials would allow for a variety of services and support. A first step in the systems change approach to support ROSC is to gather outcome data collected by monitoring and evaluation efforts and services. A second step is to conduct an inventory of recovery-focused services so that agencies could develop a comprehensive directory of recovery support services available. A final recommendation by White and colleagues is to create a state recovery resource center that would serve as a clearinghouse for recovery resources and treatment information (2008). Such a center could provide training, education, outreach, and various forms of support necessary for recovery.

A Call for the Integration of Mental Health Substance Use ROSC

Davidson outlines several perspectives, challenges, and recommendations within the ROSC movement and operationalization worth noting (Davidson et al., 2021). In 2002, Connecticut adopted a policy on promoting ROSC and called for strength, support, mastery, and regaining that lead to meaning and purpose within a broader community. Davidson's model focuses on stage agency partners, integration MHSU authorities, and community collaboration. Expanding on the ROSC models presented earlier, Davidson's model calls for ongoing recovery support through public education and prevention, outreach and engagement, active treatment and rehabilitation, and monitoring and early reintervention (2021). Within this model, the stages of recovery are priming, initiation and stabilization, management, and citizenship. One observation about this model is the last stage of recovery is **citizenship which represents an individual's connection to their rights, responsibilities, roles, and resources within a community or society** (Ponce & Rowe, 2018).

Public Health Takeaway Citizenship as an outcome is more aligned with a public health and health-equity focused approach rather than focusing on outcomes like abstinence or psychological wellbeing. Indeed, citizenship captures the intended outcome of ROSC approaches, bringing people back into their communities, to gain their rightful place.

Evaluators make recommendations, collect data, analyze data, meet with communities, and develop solid recommendations about what to do next. Karakus and colleagues conducted an Open Forum exploratory study in 2016 and identified eight big recommendations for improving the effectiveness of the US behavioral healthcare system (Karakus et al., 2017). These recommendations are based on a shared agreement that the objective of behavioral health (and I would add SU) is to deliver evidence-based services that are culturally sensitive and improve lives.

#1   Incentivize behavioral health care
#2   Provide flexibility within financing vehicles to support integration of care
#3   Promote measurement-based care and quality improvement systems (evaluation anyone)
#4   Maximize the use of shared, integrated EHRs and clinical registries
#5   Encourage workforce development around integrated methodologies
#6   Support patient and family-centered care
#7   Integrate providers of alcohol and drug abuse treatment into the patient-centered care team
#8   Protect patient confidentiality but remove barriers to sharing information within the care team

(Karakus et al., 2017)

Systems Change

We reviewed systems change and general systems theory in Chapter 2. If we apply the concept of systems change to systems that support recovery, we must recognize how systems improve capacity and service delivery to improve access, and/or quality for people in a recovery community. A public health approach to treatment and recovery requires an acknowledgement of what systems change is, and how it occurs within the context of communities and treatment programs. We will talk more about systems change and evaluation in Chapter 6. When thinking about the public health approach to evaluating treatment programs and the last step of widespread adoption of interventions, programs, and policies- this is where systems change can have the biggest impact (step 4).

Promising Practices from the Field: United States and World

Advancing Recovery is a national program funded by the Robert Wood Johnson Foundation. The overall goal of this program is to develop a new model that promotes evidence-based treatment for alcohol and drug disorders while addressing barriers to implementing treatments within systems. Components of the Advancing Recovery change model promote four conditions for change: understand customer needs, commitment from leadership, clear aim, and purpose, and supportive business case. Levers for change include financial analysis, regulatory and policy analysists, inter-organizational analysis, operations analysis, and customer impact analysis. These are supported by three supports for change, partnership between payer and providers, use of rapid change cycles, and technical assistance, coaching, and learning collaboratives (Schmidt et al., 2012). Researchers conducted a 3-year mixed-method evaluation to explore how treatment systems promoted two evidence-based practices, medication-assisted treatment (MAT) and continuing care management (Schmidt et al., 2012). Outcomes and implementation strategies from 12 state and county agencies were assessed. Using the Advancing Recovery Model, sites increased the number of patients they served with evidence-based practices and rates of adoption of MAT were higher than continuing care management.

In British Columbia (BC), Canada researchers reported on their public health response to the opioid overdose epidemic using the **cascade of care framework**. The concept of a cascade of care framework comes from HIV/AIDS (Gardner et al., 2011), HCV, and diabetes research, where the framework supports engagement in a treatment system and exploring attrition at various stages in the healing process (Piske et al., 2020). Using the cascade of care framework, researchers explored health-care utilization practices, attrition rates after diagnosis and treatment, regional differences in OUD and MAT diagnoses, and demographic characteristics of OUD patients. BC researchers assessed levels of MAT engagement and retention using administrative data from the healthcare system. They found that 71% of patients with OUD engaged with MAT, 33% were currently receiving MAT, and only 16% were retained after 1 year (Piske et al., 2020). Figure 4.3 is an example of a cascade of care framework using dummy data.

Evaluation of Bringing Recovery Supports to Scale Example

This chapter covered a ton on systems that support recovery, approaches, methods, measurement tools, concepts, recovery capital, and principles. But this is an evaluation book, about evaluation, and for evaluators. What do evaluators do and how are they tasked with evaluating elements of PRS and ROSC? This is just one example (and not my favorite but it will work).

In 2015 I led the evaluation of a Bringing Recovery Supports to Scale Project (BRSSP), the Peer-Led Organizations that Promote Best And Emerging Practices in Peer Services. Funded by SAMHSA, this project was developed to identify best practices for recovery support and training. This 1-year focused project included hiring a training coordinator, conducting a scan and asset map of existing recovery support resources, facilitating a 2-day training on recovery, advisory board meetings, development of a peer recovery support manual, strategic communications, evaluation of the training, and collaborations with chemical dependency departments, behavioral health, economic development,

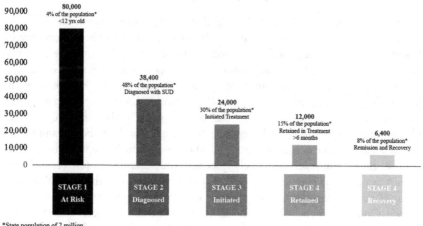

Figure 4.3 Cascade of Care Framework Example.

organizations, family, and others resulting in an implemented peer-driven culturally based model appropriate for the target population. Here is part of the evaluation report that we submitted (based on what was required) by section, question, and response. Questions are in italics.

Project Activities

Please identify key events or accomplishments during the project period (these are process related measures). The following activities were completed during the project period:

- Hired Training Coordinator
- Conducted scan and asset map of existing peer recovery support resources
- Developed an advisory board with 5 people
- Conducted 3 advisory board meetings and 12 conference calls
- Worked in a collaborative fashion to develop the workshop agenda
- Updated the Peer Recovery Support Manual
- Hosted the 2-day training October 15–16, 2015
- Conducted evaluation of the workshop using online and print formats
- Created 5 different videos as part of the training
- Collaborated with new organizations to share the culturally-appropriate peer-driven recovery model
- The strategic communications plan was developed but we did not have the time and manpower to implement the plan. In terms of this project, we had

a challenge with the website not being up and running; updating constituents was not possible via the web. We attempted to do this via Twitter, Facebook, and email communications.

Overall accomplishing these goals helped strengthen the position and visibility of the ROSC as the only Native peer-led organization in the region serving Native people. Partners and a national audience learned about the powerful stories of recovery and culturally-informed PRS approaches from this work. *Was it necessary for you to adjust your project goals as a result of what you learned in the course of implementing the project? If so, please provide additional information. If not, let us know.* We revised some of our project goals with regard to the implementation timeline and the number of people reached. For example, we initially wanted to reach a minimum of 50 people through the workshop but to date we have only reached about 35 because the videos were just recently uploaded to our YouTube account. We also had to adjust our thinking about the kinds of technology we wanted to use- we learned early on that the cost of Adobe Connect exceeded the funds available in the budget. Therefore, we partnered with another organization to host the workshop. This cost-sharing made it possible for us to build the infrastructure within our budget and it allowed us to utilize the same software as other Native organizations, tribal colleges and state partners.

Key Lessons and Strategies

- Flexibility is critical.
- The limited time period of the grant requires team members to act fast—sometimes the time it takes to bring new staff on and train them in recovery and the BRSS approach requires additional time.
- Technology costs more and takes more time that we initially thought.
- Changes in staffing and leadership impact the direction and progress of this work.
- Virtual trainings can be an effective way to reach more people at a lower cost. They are also a timeless resource—where in-person conferences last a day or two with a limited audience. Videos can reach more people over a longer period of time.
- This process helped us elevate our Peers and Peer Navigators—they were the experts, and their stories were the focus and highlight of the training. Continued efforts are needed to promote them on their healing journey.
- Lesson. Bringing education about recovery to lots of different populations is critical to begin to make recovery informed decisions that will allow for community readiness, both locally and nationally.

Evaluation, Impacts, and Changes

What steps did you take to evaluate your project?

We developed a mixed methods approach to evaluate the impact of BRSS TACS. We utilized meeting minutes, observation, videos, Peer Navigator perspectives, and Peer perspectives to evaluate the project. This was framed using a process and outcome-based evaluation approach.

The evaluation focused on the following questions:

- What has happened? What is the situation? What changes occurred for people/organizations involved?
- What were the outcomes or impacts of the program?
- Was this good? In what ways could it be better? Is this the best option? Is this cost effective? What are the strengths and weaknesses?
- What actions should be taken in the future and what changes should be made?
- How has this project had an impact on the work of your organization?

What has happened? BRSS funded the organization to host a 2-day training on PRS. This took place October 15–16, 2015. Peers shared their stories and experiences with PRS. Two officers from the City of Anonymous Motivated Addictions Program shared their approach to helping people access recovery supports. Two employers were videotaped, and they talked about their approach to being recovery informed and the importance of having recovery informed employers to best support individuals in their healing journeys. *What were the outcomes or impacts of the program?* The organization hosted the first recovery training for Native people in the region. This strengthened relationships with partners in the region and nation. People involved in the training felt empowered to help individuals in recovery. The weakness of this approach is that technology does not always work—people get frustrated when computers/systems are not set-up to view trainings. Another weakness was the multiple directions the Training Coordinator was pulled in—this took the focus off the project and diluted the project outcomes. The strengths of this approach are clear—people need to hear and see that recovery is possible. *Was this good?* This was a beneficial experience for the organization and individuals involved in PRS efforts. In the future we could improve our efforts by promoting the event early, engaging more tribal communities and chemical dependency programs while making sure they have access to video cams on their computers and address security system issues. Overall, this was cost effective—but in person meetings remain the best way to share and connect with others in recovery. *What actions should be taken in the future?* Trainings should occur monthly. The organization should utilize virtual technology as a means to promote recovery-informed employers, communities, and tribal leaders. The organization will continue to identify opportunities for Peers and Peer Navigators to share their work and recovery stories with others—making recovery possible for everyone. Online evaluation results from the training show positive impacts with responses as follows: develop new partnerships with recovery-serving individuals and organizations (67%), increase cultural relevance and sensitivity to those in recovery (65%), create and revise policies and protocols to be recovery informed (33%), and individuals felt the training validated and supports current work and practice in recovery. All participants completing the evaluation reported they attended the training to learn new information about PRS. All presenters were given above average ratings and 100% felt the training met their expectations. With regard to how they wish to be involved in future efforts, some wanted information about new funding sources, and others asked for PRS services, or opportunities to share lived recovery experiences in the future. *How has this project had an impact on the work of your organization?* This project was the first time the organization hosted a virtual training. The organization partnered with the Anonymous Corporation to utilize their equipment and office space—ultimately this resulted in improved delivery of the training and increased visibility of the BRSS efforts because the training was not in the organization's office location but in a separate building with several Native American programs. Overall this strengthened partnerships with the City of Anonymous, Community Development Program and recovery service organizations in the area. Another impact was increased knowledge about recovery and PRS among ROSC staff –working toward a goal of being recovery informed. The team finalized a Recovery Manual—this will the organization formalize future efforts and obtain funding for additional PRS training. The training and manual will be shared with non-Native PRS programs in the region with the hopes that they will incorporate culturally-responsive recovery informed PRS services.

Systems Change

Please describe any contributions your project activities may have made to the formulation of new policies, identification of new funding sources for recovery support services, or development of the recovery support services infrastructure. The organization developed a memorandum of agreement (MOA) with a treatment organization in the area to bring the Native American voice to the recovery movement in the city. New partnerships and collaborations resulting from the funding include the following: state-level partnerships, we identified 23 new potential partnerships through the state chemical dependency programs. Through BRSS the organization increased knowledge about the state's Medicaid funding for PRS. The organization also entered into an agreement with a Tribal Chemical Dependency Program to begin offering PRS in their community. The organization leveraged resources and renewed partnerships with an anonymous corporation. New partnerships with the Executive Director of State Peer Network provided several resources related to training, funding, and certifications for future consideration. National partnerships also resulted from this effort with several anonymous institutions and organizations agreeing to share resources, contacts, and listservs as a platform for sharing PRS and ROSC information from the training.

Wrap-Up

It is a wrap. In this chapter we have covered a ton of information about RSOC, recovery supports, barriers facing ROSC's, global ROSC efforts and more. One of my favorite examples from this chapter is the **Healing Forest** concept (Moore & Coyhis, 2010). I mentioned this concept to my team, students, and daughter. I have a plant forest in my bathroom, blessed with high ceilings and a ton of natural light, 15 plants call this forest their home. Every Sunday I tend to my plant forest. The Jade plant is at least 20 years old and stands strong and imposing on a 12-foot-tall ledge, ruling the forest. The Angel plant came from a start that my mom cut from Woody's Drive-in about 30 years ago. Unfortunately, my mom does not view cutting plant starts as a crime. I always feel embarrassed and pitiful when she cuts starts from yards, public places, and restaurants, as if this is something completely normal and acceptable, but that is a story for another time. The stolen Angel plant sits in the corner in an ugly plastic pot, barely visible from the ground, with long trailing leaves that produce new growth. Last Sunday while hanging from a ladder and tending to the plant forest I noticed some small bugs flying around, they were in and around Purple Queen. Recalling that I had just introduced Purple Queen to the forest two weeks ago, I knew that she could not stay. Today Purple Queen is living in an isolated room with no other plants, there is a fair amount of sun, she has a clean pot and new soil. I keep watching Purple Queen and hope she will be healthy enough to return to the plant forest. Purple Queen made me think about the Healing Forest concept. Is it enough to change Purple Queen's soil and pot? What if the bugs come back? If we apply the ROSC model described in this chapter to the Healing Forest concept, we know that even if the bugs return, there are supports, new pots, new soil, places that the plants can go, to get better, and heal.

Public Health Takeaway- What does the healing forest look like in the community or systems that you serve? Who notices the trees that are sick? What trees are sick? Why are they sick? What needs to happen in the forest so that conditions support recovery, healing, spirituality, and overall well-being? (steps 3–4).

The United States has been leading ROSC efforts for more than two decades, but recovery outcomes and well-being are less than desirable. Perhaps the lack of progress is related to the silos and the failure to fully integrate mental health and substance abuse recovery supports. Or the lack of progress may indicate we need to rethink how we conceptualize recovery and measure it. Entire books, classes, and lifetimes have been spent thinking about recovery and measuring it. This has led us down many roads, designing programs, conceptual approaches, treatment modalities, training, measures, and more. Most people (and experts) agree that there are many paths to recovery, and both individual and organizational approaches are required. I believe the concept of many paths calls for experts to step back from writing, theorizing, generalizing about treatment and recovery. We have gotten away from asking people what they think. New Zealand's work to measure recovery using just two questions could have far-reaching impacts on building individualized paths within the ROSC movement (Fitzgerald et al., 2016). New Zealand's individual measures ask people, "… are you where you want to be … and are you satisfied with your progress." It's that easy.

What if recovery is happening every day and we are just not measuring it or capturing it on the books, in the papers, funding, systems, and programs. The concept of natural recovery (to be discussed in Chapters 6–7) is an entire pandora's box of undocumented systems and paths to recovery.

Discussion Questions

1. What are the characteristics of an ROSC? What are some the barriers facing ROSC's and how might these barriers be addressed in your work as an evaluator?
2. Select one of the systems that support recovery described in this chapter (e.g., 12-Step Program). What are some potential ways that evaluators may work within these systems? Can you foresee any challenges with access, trust, bias, or stigma?
3. When you think about a public health approach to evaluating systems that support recovery (remember Chapter 2) what will be difficult? Defining the problem, identifying the cause of the problem (for example, what is supporting an ROSC and what is a barrier), determining which systems works and for whom, or ensuring widespread adoption systems that support recovery.

Resources

Recovery Oriented Systems of Care and Measures

Addiction Technology Transfer Center Network Recovery and ROSC Resources, https://attcnetwork.org/centers/global-attc/recovery-oriented-systems-care-rosc

Recovery Outcome Measures to Advance Recovery Oriented Systems of Care, https://sites.utexas.edu/mental-health-institute/files/2018/12/UT-TIEMH_Recovery-Outcome-Measures-to-Advance-Recovery-Oriented-Systems-of-Care_2018.pdf

Substance Abuse and Mental Health Services Administration ROSC Resource Guide, https://www.samhsa.gov/sites/default/files/rosc_resource_guide_book.pdf

Substance Abuse and Mental Health Services Administration Recovery Research and Evaluation Technical Expert Panel Summary Report, https://facesandvoicesofrecovery.org/wp-content/uploads/2019/06/SAMHSA-Recovery-Research-and-Evaluation-Technical-Expert-Panel-Summary-Report.pdf

Substance Abuse and Mental Health Services Administration Bringing Recovery Supports to Scale Technical Assistance Center Strategy, https://www.samhsa.gov/brss-tacs

References

Alcoholics Anonymous (n.d). The twelve steps of Alcoholics Anonymous. Retrieved November 11, 2021, from: https://www.aa.org/assets/en_US/smf-121_en.pdf

Anthony, W. A. (1993). Recovery from mental illness: The guiding vision of the mental health service system in the 1990s. *Psychosocial Rehabilitation Journal, 16*(4), 11–23. 10.1037/h0095655

Ashford, R. D., Bergman, B. G., Kelly, J. F., & Curtis, B. (2020). Systematic review: Digital recovery support services used to support substance use disorder recovery. *Human Behavior and Emerging Technologies, 2*(1), 18–32. 10.1002/hbe2.148

Association of Recovery Schools. (2021). *Find a school.* https://www.recoveryanswers.org/resource/education-based-recovery-services/

Bradshaw, N. (2019). Popular alternatives to Alcoholics Anonymous. Retrieved from: https://www.soberrecovery.com/addiction/5-popular-alternatives-to-alcoholics-anonymous

Bergman, B. G., Greene, M. C., Hoeppner, B. B., & Kelly, J. F. (2018). Expanding the reach of alcohol and other drug services: Prevalence and correlates of US adult engagement with online technology to address substance problems. *Addictive Behaviors, 87*, 74–81. 10.1016/j.addbeh.2018.06.018

Borkman, T.J., Kaskutas, L.A., Room, J., Bryan, K., & Barrows, D. (1998). An historical and developmental analysis of social model programs. *Journal of Substance Abuse Treatment, 15*(1), 7–17. 10.1016/S0740-5472(97)00244-4

Brooklyn, J. R., & Sigmon, S. C. (2017). Vermont hub-and-spoke model of care for opioid use disorder: Development, implementation, and impact. *Journal of addiction medicine, 11*(4), 286–292. 10.1097/ADM.0000000000000310

Coyhis, D., & Simonelli, R. (2005). Rebuilding native American communities. *Child welfare, 84*(2), 323–336.

Davidson, L., Rowe, M., DiLeo, P., Bellamy, C., & Delphin-Rittmon, M. (2021). Recovery-oriented systems of care: A perspective on the past, present, and future. *Alcohol Research: Current Reviews, 41*(1), 09. 10.35946/arcr.v41.1.09

Eddie, D., Hoffman, L., Vilsaint, C., Abry, A., Bergman, B., Hoeppner, B., Weinstein, C., & Kelly, J. F. (2019). Lived experience in new models of care for substance use disorder: A systematic review of peer recovery support services and recovery coaching. *Frontiers in Psychology, 10*, 1052. 10.3389/fpsyg.2019.01052

Expert-panel-05222012.pdf. (n.d.). Retrieved November 11, 2021, from https://www.samhsa.gov/sites/default/files/expert-panel-05222012.pdf

Finch, A. J., Tanner-Smith, E., Hennessy, E., & Moberg, D. P. (2018). Recovery high schools: Effect of schools supporting recovery from substance use disorders. *The American Journal of Drug and Alcohol Abuse, 44*(2), 175–184. 10.1080/00952990.2017.1354378

Galanter, M. (2007). Spirituality and recovery in 12-step programs: An empirical model. *Journal of Substance Abuse Treatment, 33*(3), 265–272. 10.1016/j.jsat.2007.04.016

Gardner, E. M., McLees, M. P., Steiner, J. F., Del Rio, C., & Burman, W. J. (2011). The spectrum of engagement in HIV care and its relevance to test-and-treat strategies for prevention of HIV infection. *Clinical Infectious Diseases: An Official Publication of the Infectious Diseases Society of America, 52*(6), 793–800. 10.1093/cid/ciq243

Granfield, R., & Cloud, W. (2001). Social context and natural recovery: The role of social capital in the resolution of drug-associated problems. *Substance Use & Misuse, 36*(11), 1543–1570. 10.1081/JA-100106963

Groshkova, T., Best, D., & White, W. (2013). The assessment of recovery capital: Properties and psychometrics of a measure of addiction recovery strengths. *Drug and Alcohol Review, 32*(2), 187–194. 10.1111/j.1465-3362.2012.00489.x

Jason, L. A., Olson, B. D., Ferrari, J. R., & Lo Sasso, A. T. (2006). Communal housing settings enhance substance abuse recovery. *American Journal of Public Health, 96*(10), 1727–1729. 10.2105/AJPH.2005.070839

Jason, L. A., Salomon-Amend, M., Guerrero, M., Bobak, T., O'Brien, J., & Soto-Nevarez, A. (2021). The emergence, role, and impact of recovery support services. *Alcohol Research: Current Reviews, 41*(1), 04. 10.35946/arcr.v41.1.04

Jury, A., & Smith, M. (2016). Measuring Recovery in adult community addiction services. *New Zealand Journal of Psychology (Online), 45*(1), 13.

Karakus, M., Ghose, S. S., Goldman, H. H., Moran, G., & Hogan, M. F. (2017). "Big eight" recommendations for improving the effectiveness of the U.S. behavioral health care system. *Psychiatric Services, 68*(3), 288–290. 10.1176/appi.ps.201500532

Kelley, A. (2021, September 8). Recovery. *Recovery.* Retrieved November 11, 2021, from https://www.allysonkelleypllc.com/post/national-recovery-month

Kemppainen, K. Kopera-Frye, J. Woodard. (2008). The medicine wheel: A versatile tool for promoting positive change in diverse contexts. *Collected Essays on Learning and Teaching,* v1 p80–84 2008. ISSN-2368-4526. Retrieved from: https://files.eric.ed.gov/fulltext/EJ1055071.pdf

Kennedy, E. S. E., & Horton, S. (2011). "Everything that I thought that they would be, they weren't:" Family systems as support and impediment to recovery. *Social Science & Medicine (1982), 73*(8), 1222–1229. 10.1016/j.socscimed.2011.07.006

McDonnell, A., MacNeill, C., Chapman, B., Gilbertson, N., Reinhardt, M., & Carreiro, S. (2021). Leveraging digital tools to support recovery from substance use disorder during the COVID-19 pandemic response. *Journal of Substance Abuse Treatment, 124,* 108226. 10.1016/j.jsat.2020.108226

Mowbray, O., Quinn, A., & Cranford, J. (2014). Social networks and alcohol use disorders: Findings from a nationally representative sample, *The American Journal of Drug and Alcohol Abuse, 40*(3), 181–186, DOI: 10.3109/00952990.2013.860984

Moore, D., & Coyhis, D. (2010). The multicultural wellbriety peer recovery support program: Two decades of community-based recovery. *Alcoholism Treatment Quarterly, 28*(3), 273–292. 10.1080/07347324.2010.488530

National Institute on Drug Abuse (2017, June 15). *Recovery.* Retrieved November 11, 2021, from https://www.drugabuse.gov/drug-topics/recovery

Neale, J., Vitoratou, S., Finch, E., Lennon, P., Mitcheson, L., Panebianco, D., Rose, D., Strang, J., Wykes, T., & Marsden, J. (2016). Development and validation of 'SURE': A patient reported outcome measure (PROM) for recovery from drug and alcohol dependence. *Drug and Alcohol Dependence, 165,* 159–167. 10.1016/j.drugalcdep.2016.06.006

Owens, M. D., & McCrady, B. S. (2014). The role of the social environment in alcohol or drug relapse of probationers recently released from jail. *Addictive Disorders & Their Treatment, 13*(4), 179–189. 10.1097/ADT.0000000000000039

Oxford House (2021). Self-run, self-supported recovery houses. Retrieved from: https://oxfordhouse.org/

Pincus, H. A., Spaeth-Rublee, B., Sara, G., Goldner, E. M., Prince, P. N., Ramanuj, P., Gaebel, W., Zielasek, J., Großimlinghaus, I., Wrigley, M., van Weeghel, J., Smith, M., Ruud, T., Mitchell, J. R., & Patton, L. (2016). A review of mental health recovery programs in selected industrialized countries. *International Journal of Mental Health Systems, 10*(1), 73. 10.1186/s13033-016-0104-4

Piske, M., Zhou, H., Min, J. E., Hongdilokkul, N., Pearce, L. A., Homayra, F., Socias, M. E., McGowan, G., & Nosyk, B. (2020). The cascade of care for opioid use disorder: A retrospective study in British Columbia, Canada. *Addiction, 115*(8), 1482–1493. 10.1111/add.14947

Polcin, D. L., Korcha, R. A., Bond, J., & Galloway, G. (2010). Sober living houses for alcohol and drug dependence: 18-month outcomes. *Journal of Substance Abuse Treatment, 38*(4), 356–365. 10.1016/j.jsat.2010.02.003

Ponce, A. N., & Rowe, M. (2018). Citizenship and community mental health care. *American Journal of Community Psychology, 61*(1–2), 22–31. 10.1002/ajcp.12218

Recovery Research Institute. (n.d.). Education-based recovery services. *Recovery Research Institute Special Topics and Resources.* Retrieved September 30, 2021, from https://www.recoveryanswers.org/resource/education-based-recovery-services/

Reif, S., Braude, L., Lyman, D. R., Dougherty, R. H., Daniels, A. S., Ghose, S. S., Salim, O., & Delphin-Rittmon, M. E. (2014). Peer recovery support for individuals with substance use disorders: Assessing the evidence. *Psychiatric Services, 65*(7), 853–861. 10.1176/appi.ps.201400047

SAMHSA (2010). Recovery-oriented systems of care resource guidebook. Retrieved November 11, 2021, from https://www.samhsa.gov/sites/default/files/rosc_resource_guide_book.pdf

SAMHSA (2012). Operationalizing Recovery-Oriented Systems. Expert Panel Meeting Report. May 22–23, 2012. https://www.samhsa.gov/sites/default/files/expert-panel-05222012.pdf

SAMHSA (2020). Recovery-oriented systems of care. Retrieved November 11, 2021, from https://www.samhsa.gov/find-help/recovery

Schmidt, L. A., Rieckmann, T., Abraham, A., Molfenter, T., Capoccia, V., Roman, P., Gustafson, D. H., & McCarty, D. (2012). Advancing recovery: Implementing evidence-based treatment for substance use disorders at the systems level. *Journal of Studies on Alcohol and Drugs, 73*(3), 413–422. https://www.ncbi.nlm.nih.gov/pmc/articles/PMC3594882/

Smith, A. (2019). Got tell it on the mountain? Recovery.org. Retrieved November 11, 2021, from https://www.recovery.org/pro/articles/the-case-for-keeping-your-recovery-off-social-media/

Sussman, S. (2010). A review of alcoholics anonymous/narcotics anonymous programs for teens. *Evaluation & the Health Professions, 33*(1), 26–55. 10.1177/0163278709356186

Stevens, M., Chubinsky, K., & Kuhn, W. (2018). Recovery outcome measures to advance recovery oriented systems of care. Texas Institute for Excellence in Mental Health, School of Social Work, University of Texas at Austin. Retrieved November 11, 2021, from https://sites.utexas.edu/mental-health-institute/files/2018/12/UT-TIEMH_Recovery-Outcome-Measures-to-Advance-Recovery-Oriented-Systems-of-Care_2018.pdf

White, M. (2008). Recovery management and recovery-oriented systems of care: Scientific rationale and promising practices. Retrieved November 11, 2021, from https://www.semanticscholar.org/paper/Recovery-management-and-recovery-oriented-systems-White/158905aae92ef779fe0a6a212dacc954b7d9a269

White, W. L., & Kurtz, E. (2008). Twelve defining moments in the history of Alcoholics Anonymous. In L. A. Kaskutas, & M. Galanter (Eds.), *Recent developments in alcoholism* (Vol. 18, pp. 37–57). Springer New York. 10.1007/978-0-387-77725-2_3

5 Examples of Evaluation Approaches for Prevention, Treatment, and Recovery

CONTENTS

DOI: 10.4324/9781003290728-5

Learning Objectives

After reading this chapter you should be able to …

1. Define five evaluation principles that advance equity and justice.
2. Describe components of treatment program evaluation timelines.
3. List the four steps to a public health program evaluation and list one example for each based on the readings provided.
4. List examples of treatment program evaluation informed by a public health approach, discuss the challenges and strengths of each.

The Approach

I believe that we do not learn how to evaluate anything by reading a book, or even taking a class. We learn evaluation by doing evaluation. It is not always easy, and when you are first starting out you will make mistakes. Mistakes are how we learn and become better evaluators. This chapter provides examples of how to evaluate various treatment programs. The first section summarizes basic evaluation principles that you may already know from your work. We discussed some of these principles in Chapter 3. The second section provides specific programs, approaches, examples, outcomes, and lessons that I learned along the way. Evaluation can be messy so get ready for a fun ride.

Principles for All Evaluators

The American Evaluation Association identified five principles for evaluators to follow when working in the field. These should be adhered to when conducting evaluations of treatment programs. You will recall these are: **Systematic Inquiry**: Evaluators conduct data-based inquiries that are thorough, methodical, and contextually relevant. **Competence**: Evaluators provide skilled professional services to stakeholders. **Integrity**: Evaluators behave with honesty and transparency in order to ensure the integrity of the evaluation. **Respect for People**: Evaluators honor the dignity, well-being, and self-worth of individuals and acknowledge the influence of culture within and across groups. **Common Good and Equity**: Evaluators strive to contribute to the common good and advancement of an equitable and just society (American Evaluation Association, 2018). In addition, evaluations must adhere to these four basic standards: utility, feasibility, propriety, and accuracy.

Program Evaluation Timelines

Evaluating a treatment program can begin at any time during planning, implementation, or completion. Evaluators may work closely with treatment programs and assist them with identifying program needs, and then finding program funding that will meet those needs. The evaluation timeline will vary based on the type of evaluation that is required, the funding agency evaluation requirements, staffing needs, program capacity, and reporting requirements.

Figure 5.1 is a timeline illustrating a linear process where the needs assessment may be completed first followed by a feasibility study and process evaluation. Outcome, impact, and cost benefit evaluations often occur at the end of a program or funding cycle. Figure 5.1 shows the intake of a participant, followed by treatment, then discharge, and follow-up at 6 and 12 months. Some programs recommend shorter follow-up periods, like 30-days post discharge and at 3 months instead of six. For example, the Substance Abuse and Mental Health Services Administration (SAMHSA) grant funded programs have follow-up periods at 3-, 6-, or 12-month time periods. These are times when program staff or evaluators must collect and report on participant outcomes using a tool like the Government Performance Results Act (GPRA). The GPRA assesses participant substance use, mental health, social connections, recovery support, and employment and education related needs.

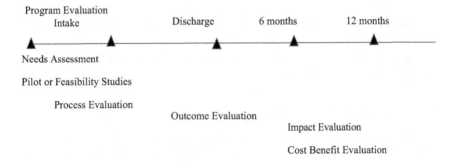

Figure 5.1 Example Program Evaluation Linear Timeline for Substance Misuse Treatment.

Table 5.1 is an example timeline submitted with a funded grant application to SAMHSA. As you can see from this timeline, the evaluator participates in several of the activities, not just collecting data. Evaluation timelines and evaluation plans are two musts for evaluators to complete early in the evaluation process.

Table 5.1 Substance Abuse Prevention Program Evaluation Timeline Example

Dates	Key Activities	Responsible Staff
Month 4-60	• Form community coalition for initial meeting • Schedule yearly events with community coalition using SPF model • Submit Quarterly Reports via SPARS	• PD, MH • CM • EV
Month 5, 10, 15, 20, 25, 30, 35, 40, 45, 50, 55, 60	• Host 1:12 community events to increase community awareness of the consequences of substance abuse	• PD, MH, CM
Month 7, 19, 31, 43, 55	• Administer CCSS to youth every 12 months	• LE, EV, MH
Month 8	• Host 1:12 community events to increase community awareness of substance abuse	• PD, MH
Month 10	• Pilot test prevention messaging campaign using resources from community	• MH, LE
Months 12	• Have three signed partnership agreements from new youth-serving organizations in the community	• PD, PC
Months 12, 24, 36, 48, 60	• Develop annual project performance assessment report highlighting achievements, barriers, adaptations, and impact from previous year using SPF model • Develop upcoming year plan based on report	• LE, EV • PD, MH, CM
Month 18	• Gauge effectiveness of prevention messaging campaign and change accordingly • Gauge community coalition members to ensure they represent 8 of the 12 sectors in prevention efforts to confirm increase in community capacity	• PD, MH, CM, LE, EV
Month 48	• Conduct CRA and compare to baseline	• MH, EV, LE
Month 60	• Goals and Objectives Completed • Final Evaluation Report with accomplishments and barriers identified for future efforts	• PD, MH, CM, LE, EV

Key activities are listed along with the primary person(s) responsible (PR) including, Project Director = PD, Mental Health Professional = MH, Coalition Members TBD = CM, Lead Epidemiologist = LE, Evaluator = EV. SPF = strategic prevention framework, CCSS = community cultural short scale, CRA = community readiness assessment.

Step 1. What Is the Problem?

This section of examples addresses the first step in a public health approach to treatment program evaluation. Here are some approaches for defining the problem in a treatment program evaluation.

Needs Assessment Treatment Program Evaluation Examples

If you are reading this text, you may have written a federally funded grant application for a substance misuse treatment program. The needs assessment process actually starts when an application or a concept is generated. For example, the first section of a grant application may require you to document the needs of the population. A recent SAMHSA grant application we developed required the following sections for a medication assisted treatment (MAT) grant. Identify your population(s) of focus and the geographic catchment area where services will be delivered. Describe the extent of the problem in the catchment area, including service gaps, and document the extent of the need (i.e., current prevalence rates or incidence data) for the population(s) of focus identified in your response. Identify the source of the data (SAMHSA, n.d.). The next section is an example of how we developed a needs assessment in response to a grant application for treatment and prevention efforts. Please note names, data, and location have changed to protect the programs and populations that we serve.

Box 5.1   Needs Assessment Example from SAMHSA Grant Application

We need more MAT qualified treatment providers; we need more families willing to support their loved ones in recovery- Treatment Program Director, 2019

Section A: Population of Focus and Statement of Need (10 points – 1 page)

1. Identify and describe your population(s) of focus and the geographic catchment area where services will be delivered.

The community is located in central Washington. With more than 2.2 million acres of land, the county has it's own governance structure—this proposal was developed by the Jones County Recovery Program. According to the 2010 US Census, there are 4,368 people that live in Jones County.

Focus Population. The proposed project will provide evidence-based services and practices for 20 clients (10 each year) with OUD and other stimulant misuse and use disorders. Participants will be adults, ages 18 and

---

over, who have OUD and other stimulant disorders. Participants will include both males and females. Most clients speak fluent English.

2. Describe the extent of the problem in the catchment area, including service gaps, and document the extent of the need (i.e., current prevalence rates or incidence data) for the population(s) of focus identified in your response to A.1. Identify the source of the data.

Published Prevalence Rates and Needs. A 2018 Survey at the University of Washington reported that opioid-related poisoning deaths are stabilizing, the national rate of poisoning deaths due to illicit and prescription opioids was 7.4 per 100,000 for Washington compared with 10.4 for the Nation. One factor contributing to OUD is that the state of Washington prescribes more opioids than the national average (711 per 1,000 persons compared with 665 per 1,000 US). According to the Washington Hospital Association 2014-2015 report, there were 31 per 00,000 prescriptions opioid-related in client discharges for Jones County, this was the second highest discharge rate in the state (Tumbleweed County reported 38 per 100,000).

Environmental Scans

Environmental scans are broad reviews of existing data (secondary data) to explore resources, services, and systems. Environmental scans may be used by evaluators to gather and review information that helps programs make strategic decisions about everything from healthcare staffing, data management, treatment modalities, expansion, policy change, and more. Some general steps involved in an environmental scan include documenting existing resources, services, and systems. Describing funding sources and existing resources, identifying policies and procedures, identifying technology resources, and describing system change and integration activities. Evaluators may conduct a needs assessment first, then move to an environmental scan an overall comprehensive plan for a treatment program. Alternatively, evaluators may complete just one of these approaches, the approach and method will vary based on resources, capacity, timeline, and needs. Table 5.2 is an example of treatment program needs assessment and environmental scan template.

Environmental Scan Example

The Canadian Centre on Substance Abuse published an environmental scan of addiction treatment indicators in Canada (Thomas, 2005). This scan identified health service delivery systems and addiction treatment data collected by providers in the country. The overall goal of the scan was to create a national addiction treatment data collection analysis system for the entire country. Authors began with a description of current efforts and reform focus areas. The next section of the scan included surveys collected across Canada and various data elements collected by the largest addiction treatment providers. Finally, the

Table 5.2 Treatment Program Needs Assessment and Environmental Scan Planning Sheet

Needs Assessment

Target and sub-populations	Risk and protective factors	Indicators, data types and elements	Data sources	
Environmental Scan				Gaps identified
Resources, systems, or services	Funding sources	Politics and public policies	Technology, research, attitudes, and interests	

Table 5.3 Example of Treatment Program Environmental Scan Data Types and Elements

Data Type	Data Elements Collected
Service data	Program type outpatient or inpatient
Client data	Demographics, name address, phone, gender, age, race, ethnicity
Substance use/gambling data	Problem substances alcohol, alcohol and other drugs, prescription drugs, illicit drugs, problem gambling
Assessment instruments used	Addiction Severity Index (ASI)

(Source: Adapted from Thomas, 2005).

scan included data systems used with addiction treatment settings and re-commendations for future national-level addiction treatment data (Thomas, 2005). Data types that may be included in a treatment program environmental scan include service data, client data, substance use or mental health data, and assessment instruments. Table 5.3 outlines data types and elements collected by the Ministry of Health and Social Services (Thomas, 2005).

Instruments Used in Needs Assessment Process

Once you know what types of needs assessment data is required, you can begin to consider different data sources.

Survey Development

You may find that a standardized survey will not meet your evaluation needs or provide a sufficient response to answer a critical evaluation question. Evaluators develop, pilot, and implement surveys all of the time. Some surveys are better than others. In 2017, I worked with a Tribal Epidemiology Center to document health priorities that would inform future program development, technical assistance, re-search, policy, advocacy, and funding efforts. We developed a survey in partnership with one community and Health Department, one senior researcher, and two college interns from the community. **Survey Pilot Phase.** We followed set criteria to pre-test the survey including the following: establish intended meaning of questions, agree upon the criteria used to judge the appropriateness of questions, select methods for assessing survey questions and pilot approach, and review and revise questions based on community context and cultural norms. The criteria used in the pilot and revision process included: no negative survey questions and double negative answers, only one question at a time, appropriate language for the community, simple questions that are grammatically correct, include local issues and possible health priorities, and questions make sense to everyone. Interns working on the project piloted the survey with five members of the target population had diverse life experiences and public health views. The survey took less than 5 minutes to complete per participant. As participants went through the survey, they asked questions and to elaborate on survey items. Interns recorded revisions based on community member feedback. **Survey Revision Phase.** Community participants pointed out several culturally-ineffective survey characteristics, which emerged as important considerations for continued survey development. The team collaborated to incorporate these recommended revisions to ensure any future data collected through the survey would be relevant for informing community-driven health agendas. This process was a back-and-forth progression to absorb community recommendations in the survey design. **Recommendations.** Pilot surveys in communities prior to implementation. This results in a more meaningful process and quality data. Cultivate partnerships between Tribal, private, and community organizations. Partnerships can lead to more culturally responsive survey methods. Seek equity and funding to support the partnership building process and the time it takes to engage community members (Fisher & Ball, 2003). **Lessons Learned.** Honor the unique language, culture, and history of communities in the survey design process. This broadens discourse to include multiple paradigms and alleviates tensions between communities and professionals. Identify key partners early in the survey development process and compensate community partners for their time and work. Interns were compensated for their time developing and piloting the survey. Community members were not compensated for completing the pilot survey, but this is recommended for future efforts. Determine what information is needed and how this information should be collected. Know community specific guidelines and protocols for collecting data. Keep the survey as short and as simple as possible. Only collect survey data if it will be used. Integrate community input into surveys through piloting. Failure to pilot surveys may result in a poorly designed survey and poor-quality data. Poor-quality data are not relevant, meaningful, or useful in addressing public health needs and priorities communities (Kelley et al., 2020; Kelley, Piccione, et al., 2019).

Administrative and Secondary Data

Administrative and secondary data are commonly used in the needs assessment process.

- Community or Program Stakeholder Survey

- Key Informant Interviews
- Community Asset Mapping
- Community or Program Stakeholder Discussions
- Prioritization Processes
- Administrative and Secondary Data

Treatment programs, public health professionals, and evaluators have been using administrative and secondary data to understand treatment needs for nearly 50 years (Kelley et al., 2020). These data, characterized as not collected by the individual using the data, is used to identify needs, and set priorities for program design and implementation. We explored some examples of secondary data sources in Chapter 3, these may include health care systems data, social services data, law enforcement data, and national data surveillance data, and other data that is not collected within a treatment program but utilized in the evaluation.

National Outcome Measures (NOMs) Data Example

One of the biggest data sources used to understand prevalence, needs, and impact of treatment programs comes from SAMHSA's NOM's mental health and substance use disorder domains. The NOMs data covers the following domains: abstinence, employment and education, crime and criminal justice involvement, stability in housing, access to services and service capacity, retention, social connectedness, perceptions of care, cost effectiveness, and the use of evidence-based practices (SAMHSA, 2019). Table 5.4 is an excerpt from a treatment program evaluation that included NOMs data. We reviewed demographic characteristics at baseline and 6-month follow-up with 65 American Indian participants involved in a treatment program (Kelley et al., 2017). Table 5.4 shows changes reported by participants involved in the treatment program.

Alcohol and drug related data sources come from a variety of places. These include death certificate data, coroner or medical examiner data, emergency department and hospital discharge data, police data, 911 call data, Emergency Medical Service data, syndromic surveillance data, Drug Enforcement Administration Automation of Reports and Consolidated Orders System data, National Survey of Drug Use and Health (NSDUH) data, National HIV Risk Behavior Survey (NHBS), Behavioral Risk Factor Surveillance System (BRFSS), Youth Risk

Table 5.4 Example of Baseline to Follow-up Changes With NOMs Survey Questions

Interview	Baseline	Follow Up	Change
Housed	15	35	133.3%
Employed (full time/part time)	16	28	75.0%
Monthly income average	$226.37	$193.75	−14.4%
Health status (very good or excellent)	18.0%	30.8%	71.1%

(Kelley et al., 2017).

Behavior Survey (YRBS), Prescription Drug Monitoring Program Data (PDMP), claims data from insurance payer claims databases or Medicare, clinical and payer data from EHRs, Health Information Exchange, or claims data, State Unintentional Drug Overdose Reporting System (SUDORS), Treatment Episode Data, (TEDS), American Association of Poison Control Center's National Poison Data System (NPDS), and more. The Resources section at the end of this chapter includes hyperlinks to find most of these data sources.

Opioid Data

There are multiple opioid-related data sources available for evaluators and treatment programs. Examples of primary opioid data could include EHR records that ask participants about their use of opiates. One example from a treatment program is, "During the past 30-days, how many days have you used opiates?" Response options are listed by the type of opiate, number of days, and the route. Opiates include Heroin, Morphine, Dialudid, Demerol, Percocet, Darvon, Codeine, Tylenol 2,3,4, or OxyContin/Oxycodone.

Addiction Severity Index (ASI)

ASI is a widely used tool used by treatment programs to guide treatment planning. The ASI is a semi-structured interview assessing both lifetime and recent (30 days prior to treatment entry) events and behaviors in seven domains (Medical, Employment, Drug, Alcohol, Legal, Family/Social, and Psychiatric). This instrument has excellent inter-rater and test-retest reliability, as well as discriminant and concurrent validity. The composite scores in each domain range from 0 (no problems) to 1 (severe problems) (Chaudhury et al., 2010). Treatment programs may review ASI baseline and follow-up scores by year to explore trends in ASI domains.

ASI responses are based on a severity rating from 0 to 9. Ratings include the following: 0–1: No imminent problem, treatment not indicated. 2–3: Slight problem; treatment may not be necessary. 4–5: Moderate problem, a treatment plan should be considered. 6–7: Considerable difficulty, begin a treatment plan. 8–9: Extreme problem, treatment is vital. ASI screening questions include the following areas and questions: **Medical.** How many days have you experienced medical problems in the past 30 days? Are you taking any prescribed medication on a regular basis for a physical problem? **Employment/Support Status.** Level of education completed? How long was your longest full-time job? How many people depend on you for the majority of their food, shelter, etc.? **Alcohol/ Drugs.** How many times in your life have you been treated for alcohol abuse? How much money would you say you spent during the past 30 days on drugs? How many days have you been treated in an outpatient setting for alcohol or drugs in the past 30 days? **Legal Status.** How many times in your life have you been arrested and charged with shoplifting or vandalism? How many times in your life have you been charged with driving while intoxicated? Are you presently awaiting charges, trial, or sentencing? **Family/Social Relationships.** Do you live with anyone who uses non-prescribed drugs? How many close friends do you have? Has anyone ever abused you? **Psychiatric Status.** How many times have you been treated for any psychological or emotional problems? Have you had a significant period of time (that was not a direct result of drug/alcohol use) in which you have experienced serious anxiety or tension?

Use of ASI Scores in Evaluation Example

Chaudry and colleagues explored ASI composite scores to predict HIV sexual- and drug-risk scores in pregnant women with drug use (Chaudhury et al., 2010). They found that the legal composite score was the only significant predictor of sexual risk scores, where a 1 point standard deviation increase in legal composite scores, increased sexual risk by 24% (Chaudhury et al., 2010). Table 5.5 is an example of ASI scores over a 4-year period at one treatment center. You can see from this table that employment was largest problem.

Example of Program Data and YRBSS Data

Evaluators often utilize primary and secondary data to determine value and impact. This example is an excerpt of results from an evaluation that I led comparing tribal program substance use norms and YRBSS data. This was part of a larger evaluation of a culturally-based substance misuse prevention program (Kelley et al., 2019; Kelley et al., 2020). Our goal was to compare prevalence data and norms of the program participants with data from the YRBSS to determine if there were notable differences in substance use. Table 5.6 presents data by youth on or near a Reservation (92.5% of program youth) relative to an urban setting (6.2%). Binge drinking (6.3% vs. 15.2% YRBSS) and past 30 day marijuana use (20.1% vs. 39.8% YRBSS) were substantially lower for program reservation youth relative to the Montana YRBSS findings, while higher for binge drinking (23.8% vs. 17.8% YRBSS urban) and comparable for marijuana use (22.7% vs. 23.7% YRBSS urban) for youth in an urban setting (Kelley et al., 2020). (Table 5.6)

Table 5.5 ASI Composite Domains and Scores

ASI Domain	Composite ASI Scores
Medical	.32
Employment	.83
Alcohol	.04
Drug	.28
Legal	.18
Relationship	.25
Psychiatric	.19

Table 5.6 Example of Substance Use Norms from Prevention Program and YRBSS Data Comparison Urban vs. Reservation

Measure	Program (n = 711)	T Program Tribe 1 (n = 203)	YRBSS All Montana HS Weighted %
Substance use			
Any Illegal drug use, past 30 days (p30)	104/693, 15.0%	36/197, 18.3%	n/a
Any days 5+ alcoholic drinks, p30	52/700, 7.4%	16/201, 8.0%	16.8%
Any marijuana use, p30	143/699, 20.5%	54/196, 27.6%	21.1%
Any synthetic marijuana use, p30	22/697, 3.2%	11/195, 5.6%	6.5% (life)
Any prescription drug misuse, p30	23/696, 3.3%	7/194, 3.6%	12.8% (life)
Any meth use, p30	6/696, 0.9%	2/194, 1.0%	2.4% (life)
Any other illegal drugs (LSD, ecstasy)	13/697, 1.9%	4/195, 2.0%	4.3% (life; e)
Any inhalants/sniffing use, p30	22/696, 3.2%	2/195, 1.0%	8.0% (life)
Norms			
Risk of harm drink 5+ drinks per week			
No Risk	62 (8.7)	22 (10.8)	n/a
Slight Risk	74 (10.4)	19 (9.4)	
Moderate Risk	199 (28.0)	39 (19.2)	
Great Risk	239 (33.6)	66 (32.5)	
Don't know	110 (15.5)	53 (26.1)	
missing	27 (3.8)	4 (2.0)	

(Source: Kelley et al., 2020).

Evaluation Plan for Drug Court Example

The first step in any evaluation is developing an evaluation plan. Sometimes these are required by funding agencies, and other times they are required for internal purposes. Even if they are not required, complete one. It will help you navigate the complexities of working in a treatment program setting and stay focused on the task at hand, determining what is effective, what is not, and how to promote equity and justice through public health informed evaluation. Here are some components of an evaluation plan we recently completed for a SAMHSA funded drug court grant implemented by a treatment program.

Introduction- include the location, demographic characteristics, culture, and any prevalence of need data that relate to the program focus.

Target population- list the inclusion criteria for the target population, for example they may be adults assisted with moderate to severe SUD at risk for re-offending

Staff- include the individuals within the program that will be involved in the implementation and evaluation of the effort

Purpose- describe the aims of the project, for example improving treatment outcomes among adults ages 18 and older through expanded evidence-based treatment services.

Goals and objectives- list the overall goals and objectives from the funded grant application. List the reasons for the evaluation, these may be to assess progress, support development and implementation of outcome tracking measures, provide systematic feedback, or document the value of the project on desired outcomes.

Evaluation standards- list which standards you will follow, within a community, treatment center, AEA guidelines, community guidelines, or other

Data collection- list how data will be collected, pay attention to population standards and vulnerabilities, most are considered vulnerable.

Evaluation framework-list steps that you will use to implement the evaluation. These may be engage community, focus the evaluation, collect information, analyze data, interpret data, and share information/findings.

Evaluation design- this may include the type (see Chapter 3) and formative, summative, or randomized experimental, non-experimental, or other designs.

Theoretical Frame- discuss the Theory of Change (ToC) and how the selected treatment strategy will lead to immediate, intermediate, and the program/community long term vision.

Outcome measures- list outcome measures of interest, these may be directly tied to funding agency requirements, for example maintenance of abstinence or reduction in substance use among clients receiving services. Include the data type, source, and frequency.

Data sources- list all data sources that may be utilized in the evaluation.

Create a tracking matrix- list evaluation aims, program components, tasks, expected outcomes, measures or frequencies, and the analyze approach used. Table 5.7 is an example of a tracking matrix from a drug court evaluation plan.

Interpretation- describe how evaluation results will be co-interpreted with stakeholders, admin staff, and clients.

Reporting plan- discuss the types of reports, requirements, frequency, and staff responsible for completing reports.

Dissemination plan- describe the evaluation reporting dissemination medium, frequency, and staff responsible for dissemination.

Use of findings- describe the groups that are most likely to use findings from the evaluation. For example, list the user of findings, what they may need or want to know, and potential uses.

Anticipating challenges and solutions- list potential challenges you may encounter when implementing the evaluation and potential solutions. For example, COVID-19 has been a significant challenge and evaluation teams are not able to travel to communities to meet in person with stakeholders. A potential solution is to use virtual technologies, weekly meetings, and rapid check-ins to build connection and rapport.

Evaluation team- list the roles and responsibilities of all evaluation team members.

Table 5.7 Tracking Matrix Example from SAMHSA-Funded Drug Court Evaluation Plan. Aim 2: To Assess the Effectiveness of the SUD Project on Sobriety and Well-Being

Program Component	Program Tasks	Expected Outcome	Measure	Analytic Approach
30 individuals participating in program	Identify, screen, refer, and provides support for OUD/SUD	30 individuals enter program, 15 complete/ sobriety	GPRA data, client data, CMS, program admin data	T-test baseline and follow-up, Descriptive statistics.
Evidence based and trauma informed curriculum	Develop and employ for expansion of services	30 individuals participate in evidence based and trauma informed curriculum to increase personal and social functioning and well-being	GPRA data, client data, CMS, admin data, client surveys and interviews	Descriptive statistics, mixed-methods, qualitative analysis

A public health focused evaluation approach requires evaluators to build relationships with programs and communities, while offering skills and support at various phases in the evaluation process. Evaluators may collaborate with communities to gather information and data. Evaluators may help programs and communities establish priorities for evaluation. Evaluators rarely work alone. Program staff, advisory board members, state, and federal agencies, tribal or state leaders, community members, professionals, and individuals with the lived experiences of recovery may be involved in the evaluation process (from the needs assessment and priority setting stage to implementing an evaluation and disseminating results). This next section highlights examples of instruments, timelines, analytic processes, and findings from several treatment program evaluations.

Step 2. What Is the Cause?

This section provides examples of risk and protective factors captured within a treatment program evaluation.

Application of a Logic Framework to Evaluate Social Determinants of Health (SDOH) Interventions

Building on the theory of change and logic models presented earlier in this text, Coughlin and colleagues designed an RCT to explore the effectiveness of an SDOH intervention aimed at African American patients in a clinical setting (Coughlin et al., 2019). Authors designed this intervention recognizing the SDOH present and integrated community resources with patient SDOH needs. Coughlin and colleagues present a logic model framework with intervention elements, mediator variables, and outcome variables that could be replicated in treatment program evaluation settings. Potential **targets for SDOH intervention** include decreased food insecurity, increased employment, increased opportunities for education, decreased substandard housing, social support, and social networks. **Primary and secondary outcomes** that authors identified based on their preliminary model and existing research include reduced emergency department (ED) visits, reduced hospitalizations, and improved patient satisfaction with primary care, improved chronic disease indicators, completion of preventive services such as mammograms, colorectal cancer screening, and immunizations, improved self-reported overall health, improved physical and mental health, reduced "no show" rates in primary care clinics, and overall lower health care costs (Coughlin et al., 2019).

Social Determinants of Health Instrument Example

SDOH continue to be one of the most widely promoted public health topics, yet treatment programs rarely incorporate SDOH into their evaluation plans or outcomes (Pinto et al., 2016), Table 5.8. Pinto and colleagues developed this 14-item questionnaire which has been translated into more than 13 languages throughout the globe.

Table 5.8 Social Determinants of Health Focused Screening Questions

Question	Response Options	SDOH Domain
1. What language would you feel most comfortable speaking in with your health care provider?	Various languages	Language is a key determinant of health; treatment programs must address language gaps and address poor access and treatment among individuals having a first language that is not English
2. How would you rate your ability to speak and understand English?	Very well, well, not well, not at all, unsure, prefer n/a, don't know	Treatment programs must address the gap of poor access to treatment and having a first language that is not English
3. In what language would you prefer to read health care information?	Various languages	Non-English speaking clients are at risk for adverse drug reactions due to reduced treatment comprehension and more likely to be unsatisfied with providers when they do not speak the same language

(Continued)

Table 5.8 (Continued)

Question	Response Options	SDOH Domain
4. Were you born in _____? If no, what year did you arrive in _____?	Yes or no Year	Immigrants report worse health outcomes, discrimination, and challenges accessing treatment
5. In what year were you born?	Year	Health and quality of life decreases with age
6. Which of the following best describes your race? Check one.	List of potential races	Racialized groups experience greater health disparities and inequities
7. What is your religious or spiritual affiliation?	List of potential affiliations	Treatment programs must be sensitive to the spiritual and religious practices of clients
8. Do you have any of the following disabilities?	List of potential disabilities	Certain intellectual disabilities are related to increased mortality, psychotropic medications may be misuses
9. What is your gender?	Female, male, trans, intersex, prefer n/a, don't know	Trans and intersex populations experience dissemination and stigma when accessing treatment programs
10. What is your sexual orientation?	Gay, lesbian, bisexual, two-spirit, queer other, prefer n/a, don't know	LGBTQ+ individuals experience negative encounters in treatment settings
11. What was your total family income before taxes last year?	Range of values from $0 to >$150,000	Low income groups are less liked to access treatment
12. How many people does this income support?	A number	Low income groups are more likely to die from conditions that can be prevented
13. What type of housing do you live in?	Own, rent, boarding, jail, homeless, group home, shelter, hostel, supportive housing, other, prefer n/a, don't know	Homeless populations experience poor health status and discrimination when accessing treatment
In general, would you say your health is…	Excellent, very good, good, fair, poor	Perceived health is a consideration for treatment and recovery planning

(Adapted from Pinto et al., 2016).

Application of Socioecological Model Evaluation Example

In Chapter 2 we reviewed the ecology of human development and nested systems based on Brofenbrenner's work (1979). Rogers and colleagues advocate for an ecological approach to understanding, treating, and evaluating treatment programs that address the current opioid epidemic (2018), Box 5.2.

Box 5.2　Ecological Framework that Supports Treatment Systems for Evaluators to Consider

Individual- Addiction, relationships, physical, and psychological symptoms, employment

Microsystem- Family, treatment community, friendships, professional relationships

Mesosystem- Addiction and pain treatment, drug dealers, users, local social networks, family and treatment community

Ecosystem- Drug trade and community, health insurance, long term treatment access, local community and government resources

Macrosystem- Rural economic and existential crisis, healthcare trends, pharmaceutical influences, insurance guidelines, attitudes about addiction

Chronosystem- Ages and development, educational and economic trends
(Bronfenbrenner, 1979; Rogers et al., 2018)

Step 3. What Works and for Whom?

This section includes examples of evaluation designs, drug court treatment program plans, and SAMHSA Opioid Response Process Measures and Evaluation Example.

These measures are similar to other program evaluations and may include numbers of people trained, educated, activities, meetings, services, referrals, follow-ups, length of time that individuals receive services, number and length of stays for physical health, mental health, or in criminal justice system/jail (Rural Health Information Hub, n.d.). Here are some examples of process measures from a SAMHSA Opioid Response Program Evaluation.

- Strategic plan. Was a new plan developed or an existing plan updated? How did the plan guide efforts? Did the plan include the mission and vision of the organization?
- Workforce development. What types of activities, evidence-based practices, curriculum, and trainings occurred? What types of participants were trained (social workers, families, justice system workers, others).
- Prevention. What types of activities were implemented, what evidence-based practices were used, how many people were reached?
- Treatment. What types of services were offered to clients? What evidence-based practices were used? How many encounters occurred during the program or treatment period? What types of medications were offered? Was MAT provided? How many unduplicated individuals received services or were treated by the program?

- Recovery support services. What types of support services were offered? For example, assistance with transportation, GED completion, court advocacy, financial planning, one-on-one support, sober activity engagement, and groups. What evidence-based practices were used? How many encounters occurred and what type of encounter was it? How many people received recovery support services?
- Treatment costs. How many individuals received financial assistance and what type of assistance did they receive? For example, travel costs or reimbursements, payment for inpatient or outpatient treatment, incentives, or others.
- Transitional assistance. How many individuals received transitional assistance from the program? What type of assistance did they receive?

Treatment Program Implementation Evaluation Examples

I work with several recovery programs that have grant funding from SAMHSA to address AUD, OUD, stimulant use, and drug/alcohol abuse. The evaluation focuses on change from before or baseline (when a participant is just starting) and after a period of time. The period of time varies and could be a week, month, 6 months, 3 months, 6 months, or 12 months.

Earlier in this chapter, we reviewed a program evaluation timeline for substance misuse treatment (see Figure 5.1). In Box 5.3, I demonstrate the number of clients served where the program evaluation or intake counts as baseline, and 6 months marks program completion.

Box 5.3   Example of Treatment Program Evaluation at Intake and Completion

A total of 422 clients completed the intake data collection; of these, 214 (51%) completed a 6-month follow-up. Overall, 58% of the sample were female with an average age of 37.6 years ($SD = 9.9$) and average monthly income of \$690 ($SD = \$2,984$) at intake. Slightly more than half were recruited from the urban #1 community location (54%), followed by reservation #2 (17%), urban #2 (16%), and the remaining three communities (13%). Seventy percent of the sample reported some past violence or trauma. Past month substance use days was extremely low (<.24 days) for the overall sample, and among both completers and non-completers.

Intake (N = 422)   Discharge (n = 208)   6 months (n = 214)
▲   ▲   ▲

Adapted from: (Kelley et al., 2021).

Alternative Pain Management Treatment Program Instrument Example

Individuals who experience chronic pain are often prescribed opioids for the management of chronic musculoskeletal pain. Overprescribing and a lack of patient monitoring by providers have led to opioid addiction, overdoses, and adverse effects to the bladder and immune system (Lee & Jo, 2019). Some treatment programs are implementing alternative pain management interventions like acupuncture to address OUD (Baker & Chang, 2016). Box 5.4 is an example of a data collection instrument from a treatment program offering acupuncture to clients with OUD.

Box 5.4   Client Pre and Post Acupuncture Treatment Surveys

Pre-Survey

We want to know more about you. Please take a minute to complete this form. Information will be used to design and implement future alternative pain management and wellness sessions. Contact Jess Jones at 123-45-6789 or visit our website at www.programnamehere.com for more information.

1. Have you ever been to an acupuncturist? Yes No
2. What are the reasons that you are here to receive treatment? (select all that apply).

   ○ Alternative to taking pain medication
   ○ Chronic back or neck pain
   ○ Headache relief
   ○ Better sleep
   ○ Stress relief
   ○ Depression and anxiety
   ○ Blood pressure normalization
   ○ Detox
   ○ Other:_____

3. Do you think that the acupuncture sessions will be helpful? Yes No Not Sure
4. How do you think that participation in the acupuncture session(s) will impact you? (select all that apply).

   ○ I will take fewer prescription medications
   ○ I will know more about alternative pain management strategies

---

- ○ I will be more hopeful about my overall health and wellness
- ○ I will feel like there are more resources in my community to help me
- ○ I will be more confident in my sobriety
- ○ I will feel like I belong
- ○ Other _____

Initials of Participant Here_____

Post-Acupuncture Survey

1. How many acupuncture sessions did you attend? _____
   _____

2. Have you ever received acupuncture, before the sessions at ESRP? Yes No

3. If the program did not offer acupuncture sessions, would you have gone to an acupuncturist on your own? Yes No Not Sure

4. What are the reasons that you attended acupuncture session (s)? (select all that apply).

   - ○ Alternative to taking pain medication
   - ○ Chronic back or neck pain
   - ○ Headache relief
   - ○ Better sleep
   - ○ Stress relief
   - ○ Depression and anxiety
   - ○ Detox
   - ○ Blood pressure normalization
   - ○ Other_____

5. Were the acupuncture sessions helpful? Yes No Not Sure

6. Using a scale from 1 to 10, please rate your health BEFORE attending acupuncture sessions and AFTER.
   1 is Very Poor Health and 10 is Very Good Health

	Health Before	*Health After*	N/A
Example of how to select a score.	①2 3 4 5 6 7 8 9 10	1 2 3 4 ⑤ 6 7 8 9 10	
Physical health	1 2 3 4 5 6 7 8 9 10	1 2 3 4 5 6 7 8 9 10	
Spiritual health	1 2 3 4 5 6 7 8 9 10	1 2 3 4 5 6 7 8 9 10	
Emotional health	1 2 3 4 5 6 7 8 9 10	1 2 3 4 5 6 7 8 9 10	
Mental health	1 2 3 4 5 6 7 8 9 10	1 2 3 4 5 6 7 8 9 10	

7. How did participation in the acupuncture session(s) impact you? (select all that apply).

   - ○ I take fewer prescription medications

- ○ I know more about alternative pain management strategies
- ○ I am more hopeful about my overall health and wellness
- ○ I feel like there are more resources in my community to help me
- ○ I am more confident in my sobriety
- ○ I feel like I belong
- ○ Other _____

8. Do you have any suggestions on how to improve future acupuncture sessions?
   Initials of Participant Here_____

Surveys were co-created between the evaluator, individuals with the lived experience of recovery, and the clinical director. **Paper surveys were administered** to clients before they started their first acupuncture session and after their last acupuncture session (8 weeks later). Clients attended sessions once per week for 60 minutes. A local evaluation intern collected surveys and entered them into Excel, 100 people completed the pre survey and 50 people completed the post survey (50% completion rate). **Descriptive statistics and basic frequency counts** were used to document reasons for attending acupuncture sessions, if they were helpful or thought they would be, and mean differences in self-reported health pre to post session. Only matched pair data (meaning individuals that completed the pre and post survey) were used in the evaluation. Clients reported in the baseline how they thought sessions would impact them, and at post, reported how sessions impacted them. Descriptive statistics including percentages for each statement were summarized and compared by response option. **Results** show that self-reported wellness scores improved from pre to post, reasons for attending sessions changed from pre to post, session impacts also changed from pre to post where individuals feel more hopeful about their overall health and wellness at post, and that was the greatest impact.

A **limitation** of this survey is that it is based on self-report data, not all participants that completed the pre survey completed the post, and social desirability bias may contribute to more favorable responses at post. Even with these limitations clients felt the sessions relieved stress and addressed chronic pain.

Education and Training Program Evaluation Example

The Food and Drug Administration offers qualified practitioners the ability to apply for a buprenorphine waiver. Waivers allow providers to prescribe buprenorphine for the treatment of OUD. A key barrier in the implementation of MAT is the limited availability of MAT providers. Kunins and colleagues developed a buprenorphine education and training curriculum, BupEd with primary care residency program participants (Kunins et al., 2013). BupEd included didactic sessions, motivational interviews, monthly case meetings, and supervised clinical experiences providing buprenorphine treatment. Kunins and colleagues evaluated BupEd outcomes, assessed the residents' delivery of buprenorphine treatment during residence, after residence, and the retention of patients treated by residents compared with attending physicians. Over a 3-year period, 2006 to 2009, 71 residents completed the BupEd program and treated 279 patients with buprenorphine. Of the residents that completed BupEd, 27.5% received a buprenorphine waiver and 17.5% prescribed buprenorphine. Treatment retention among patients was similar among residents and attending physicians. Findings suggest that BupEd is a feasible model that prepares physicians to treat OUD.

Treatment Program Client Satisfaction Evaluation Example

The Client Satisfaction Questionnaire-8 is a standardized tool used widely across treatment program settings. Kelly and colleagues assessed the psychometric properties of this tool in 1,378 residential substance abuse treatment clients located in Australia (Kelly et al., 2018). They report that the CSQ-8 is appropriate for residential substance abuse treatment settings and recommend future research to explore how changes in client characteristics are associated with outcome measures, retention, and recovery. Table 5.9 is an example of CSQ-8 questions with Likert type ratings, and how to calculate response scores.

Social Media Campaign Evaluation Example

We work with a recovery program to promote marketing techniques to disseminate messages about recovery, healing, hope, and treatment. Our work targets members of the community, youth and families of all ages, and people who access various forms of media (print, online, radio, other). Building on our review of logic models in Chapter 3, this example includes the structure/program elements, process, and outcome. Critical evaluation questions relating to the structure and program elements are: What is the nature of program messaging? Who is the target audience? Are the messages consistent with the health communication evidence and literacy approaches? Are the messages effective? Is the approach sustainable? Critical process questions include: What is the reach of the social media campaign? What is the frequency of message exposure? Critical evaluation questions about outcomes include: What are the short and long term outcomes of the social media campaign? Examples of short term outcomes may be improved awareness, knowledge, beliefs, ideas, and behaviors about substance abuse and mental health. Long term outcomes could be changes in attitudes, discriminatory practices, stigmatization, and increased utilization of treatment program services. The evaluation design is mixed methods because we

Table 5.9 Example of the CSQ-8 and Response Options

Questionnaire Item	Mean (Standard Deviation)	4	3	2	1
Example of how to report response scores	3.18 (0.51)	27.4% Excellent	62.8% Good	9.8% Fair	0% Poor
How would you rate the quality of service you received?		Excellent	Good	Fair	Poor
Did you get the kind of service you wanted?		Yes, definitely	Yes, generally	No, not at all	No, definitely not
To what extent has our service met your needs?		Almost all met	Most me	Only a few met	None met
If a friend were in need of similar help would you recommend our services?		Yes, definitely	Yes, I think so	No, I don't think so	Definitely not
How satisfied were you with the amount of help you received?		Very satisfied	Mostly satisfied	Indifferent	Quite dissatisfied
Have the services you received help you to deal more effectively with your problems		Yes, a great deal	Yes, somewhat	No, did not help	No, made it worse
In an overall sense, how satisfied are you with the services you have received		Very satisfied	Mostly satisfied	Indifferent	Quite dissatisfied
If you were seeking help again, would you come back to our services?		Yes, definitely	Yes, I think so	No, I don't think so	Definitely not

use quantitative data from social media analytics (frequencies) and qualitative data from social media content and responses. We track information about the reach of social media activities monthly and annually. Our goal in evaluating social media efforts is to capture who we are targeting, who we are missing, and the kinds of content that receives the most likes, reads, or views. We report results monthly to the treatment program and annually to the funding agency. Results are also used to improve content, promote messages and events, and reach more people in recovery.

Step 4. How Do You Do It?

This section is what we want to know. What is effective? How do evaluators and treatment programs promote the widespread adoption of treatments that work?

Treatment Program Cost Evaluation Example

Earlier in this text we discussed Cost Benefit Evaluations (CBAs) and Cost Effectiveness Assessments (CEAs). Below is an example of a CBA for one treatment program using an adapted version of the "social planner" perspective where all costs and benefits are included, regardless of the party to whom they accrue. Ettner and colleagues used a **social planner perspective** and estimated the total cost of client treatment by multiplying the number of days in each treatment modality by the average per diem cost of the modality and adding up the costs across all modalities used (2006). The number of days in treatment was calculated by subtracting the date of admission from the date of discharge and adding one, i.e., clients admitted and discharged on the same day were assigned an episode length of one day. To estimate average per diem costs of treatment, the total costs of each program were divided by the total number of client-days served by that program. Both weighted and unweighted average per diem treatment costs were calculated. On a per diem basis, outpatient treatment was the least expensive modality and residential treatment was the most expensive. The unweighted mean per diem costs was $13.62 (SD = $2.40) for methadone maintenance, $12.08 (SD = $14.70) for outpatient treatment, and $81.70 (SD = $60.68) for residential treatment. The average cost of treatment over the 9 months postbaseline was $1,583 ($3,336 unweighted) and the corresponding benefits were $11,487 (CI = $9,784, $13,180), for a benefit–cost ratio of more than 7:1, or 3:1 using unweighted costs. For clients whose initial treatment modality was outpatient or residential, the average treatment costs were $838 and $2,791, respectively ($1,505 and $6,745 unweighted). Compared with es-timated benefits of $9,049 and $16,257, benefit–cost ratios were about 11:1 and 6:1 (6:1 and 2:1 using the unweighted costs) (Ettner et al., 2006).

In Ettner's example their unweighted cost ratio was more than 7:1 and this is consistent with other CBAs reported in other studies and reports (Recovery Centers of America, n.d.). Depending on the level of evaluation and specificity required in your CBA or CEA, you may also consider a cost benefit ratio using the model 7:1 model where for every dollar spent on treatment saves $4 in healthcare costs and $7 in law enforcement and other criminal justice costs.

Behavioral Health and Substance Misuse Needs Assessment Example

Evaluators may work with program staff and stakeholders to conduct needs assessments. Needs assessments involve compiling data, defining the population and sub-population, and selecting indicators that represent need. We recently completed a behavioral health and substance misuse needs assessment in one US location significantly impacted by hurricanes. This 12-month process involved multiple stakeholders, researchers, evaluators, and behavioral health professionals. We worked with this diverse group to create a comprehensive assessment process to answer these three aims:

Aim 1: Describe what is known about the mental and behavioral health needs of the population post-2017 hurricanes.

Aim 2: Identify topics related to preparedness for future hurricanes.

Aim 3: Identify any mental and behavioral health data collection systems in the area post-2017 hurricanes.

We created an online assessment to collect community perspectives regarding the behavioral health needs of residents after the 2017 hurricane season. Some assessment questions focused on the 2017 – 2019 time period to learn more about the kinds of services that are needed after a hurricane and how to improve public health services in the future. The assessment was conducted using Qualtrics, an online survey platform. Public information officers also shared the information with other agencies and organizations in the area. The local contact sent an email invitation to their listserv that included information about the purpose of the assessment, the chance to win a $50 Visa gift card, and contact information for the agency and evaluation team. The consultant team developed the assessment after reviewing the 2019 National Survey of Drug Use and Health, 2018 Behavioral Risk Factor Surveillance System Survey, 2018 Associated Press NORC Survey, and SAMHSA's Behavioral Health Treatment Needs Assessment Toolkit. The 26-question assessment included demographic information, perceptions of mental and behavioral health needs, and recommendations for the response to future hurricanes. All questions and response options were then reviewed and revised by the team using an iterative process, with attention to norms, language, and culture. **Online Assessment Analytic Process.** Online assessment data from Qualtrics was downloaded into an Excel file. Quantitative data analyses were conducted by the consultant team using simple descriptive statistics and frequency counts. Qualitative data from online assessment text responses were reviewed by the consultant team using modified content analysis methods which call for transcribing, identifying codes, coding similar responses, and summarizing data. Online assessment data were combined with Key Informant Interview (KII) data. The process of interviewing and analyzing KII data is described next. **Key Informant Interview Methods.** Purposive sampling was used to identify and recruit Key Informant Interviewees (KIIs) (Palinkas et al., 2015). The sampling frame consisted of former and current employees. The local partner contacted potential interviewees, provided an overview of the project, and asked them to contact the evaluation team to set up an interview time if they were interested in participating. The potential participant was then contacted by phone or email to schedule the interview. Interviews began with the review of the consent form with verbal consent obtained before continuing with the interview. The consultant team conducted the interviews via Zoom from November 1 to December 23, 2020. Each interviewee was offered a $50 gift card to compensate them for their time. Of the eight people identified by the partner, six agreed to be interviewed. **Interview Guide Design.** The team developed a 7-question semi-structured interview guide with a focus on individual, family, community, and systems level needs as they relate to gaps in services, surveillance, policy, and preparedness for future hurricanes in the location. **Transcription procedures.** Recordings were transcribed by the consultant team and then cross-checked by a separate team member. All identifying information that could be linked to informants was removed and interviewees were assigned a unique identification number. **Theoretical Frame and Analytic Process.** Sociocultural and healthcare factors were explored at the individual, household, and community level using an adapted version of the critical medical ecological model (De Ver Dye et al., 2020; McLeroy et al., 1988). This model was appropriate because it focused on multi-level factors across sociocultural and healthcare domains. Coding of interview text was based on these typologies and identifying gaps and strengths related to the mental and behavioral health needs at the individual, household, and community level. The team utilized the six-stage Framework Method to guide the analysis process: (1) familiarization, (2) identifying a thematic framework (sociocultural and healthcare factors informed by the medical ecological model), (3) indexing, (4) charting, (5) mapping, and (6) interpretation (Bryman & Burgess, 1994). **Data analysis** was completed using hand-coding methods and NVivo version 12.0. Three major subject charts were developed to further analyze patterns in the data. Mapping involved examining core characteristics of the data and interpreting the data according to the subject charts and sociocultural and healthcare factors.

The needs assessment example presented above provided detailed information using primary data to explore three specific aims, (1) what is known about mental and behavioral health needs of the population post-2017 hurricanes, (2) what are the preparedness topics for future hurricanes, and (3) what are the behavioral health data collection systems available post-2017 hurricanes. The overall goal of this needs assessment was to document needs, populations, and indicators. Through evaluation and data collection, this was achieved.

Prevention Program Evaluation Example

Youth substance is a significant public health problem. American Indian youth are placed at higher risk for substance use due to social inequalities like exposure to violence, discrimination, and historical and present trauma. This example focuses on the first 3-years of a SAMSHA funded community-based prevention program based on the Strategic Prevention Framework and the Partnerships for Success Framework. A community-based participatory research (CBPR) approach guided the evaluation. Elders, community members, and the evaluator led the overall evaluation effort. **Setting.** The program included five reservation communities and one urban location in the Rocky Mountain Region. **Evaluation design.** Quasi-experimental Design with Intervention and Treatment Group (see Chapter 3). **Questions.** Was the prevention program effective? Did community involvement increase over time? Are there differences in AI youth who participate in culturally-based activities (intervention group) compared with AI youth who do not (non-intervention group). **Three evaluation outcomes** guided the evaluation: lower substance use among youth, increased readiness to support prevention and increased number of community members reached through culturally-based prevention efforts. **Indicators** for these outcomes were the percentage of youth who do not use illegal substances, community readiness scores, and the number of community members reached by activity and year. **Evaluation tools** included a 16-item survey for intervention and non-intervention groups, CRA (Community Readiness Assessment) interviews, and site tracking matrices. Tools came from community developed and standardized instruments to measure self-esteem, social support, substance use, and family communication. Data were verified by survey results, CRA transcripts and codes, and quarterly reports submitted to the evaluation team. This summary presents the results from the third question, "Are there differences in AI youth who participate in culturally-based activities (intervention group) compared with those who do not?" **Analysis.** One-way ANOVAs were used to examine differences between groups. The mean scores for social support differed significantly at the 5% level: $F (1,522) = 15.81$; $p = .00$ where social support was higher among intervention youth than non-intervention youth. Similarly, the mean scores for community connections differed significantly at the 5% level: $F (1,545) = 4.92$; $p = .027$. Community connections were higher among intervention youth than non-intervention youth. Results suggest that youth who participate in cultural activities may have greater social support and greater connections to their community. Both are protective factors that may delay or prevent substance use. **Limitations.** The purposive sampling approach may contribute to selection bias, social desirability may present bias for self-report questions, and non-intervention group youth may have participated in other cultural activities not reported within the current program (Kelley et al., 2019).

Peer Recovery Support Evaluation Example

We completed an evaluation of a peer recovery support program 2 years ago. The overall goals of this program were to decrease substance use in participants. Certified peer recovery support specialists met weekly with program participants and provided a variety of support. We developed two critical evaluation questions: 1) How does peer recovery support help people in recovery? and 2) Why is peer recovery support effective?

Study design-A descriptive qualitative case study design allowed us to explore the essence of peer recovery support. Consistent with qualitative study designs, our approach was grounded in an interpretivist position, meaning we were most concerned about the experience of recovery and understanding peer perspectives about peer recovery support. The case study approach was appropriate because we were interested in the phenomenon of PRS based on real-life contexts.

Data collection- Key informants were selected by the lead peer mentor and peer using convenience sampling methods. Criteria for selection of informants was participation in the program for at least 6-months and evidence that they utilized peer recovery support services provided. All were located in two states. Other demographic information was not collected due to the sensitive nature of recovery and the small number of peers interviewed. Qualitative semi-structured interviews were conducted with six peers to explore the perceptions and lived experiences of recovery. Individuals were interviewed by a peer who worked closely with the program evaluator. The peer mentor identified a peer to conduct interviews with other peers. The evaluator trained the peer in qualitative data collection techniques and how to conduct interviews. The peer also received payment for their work. Together the peer mentor, peer, and evaluator formulated an interview guide. Interviews began with peers providing verbal consent to participate in the evaluation. Responses were transcribed using a pen and paper, and text message. All participants received a $50 gift card to compensate them for their time. These interviews served as the data source for this evaluation. IRB review and approval of this evaluation was conducted prior to data collection. Interview guides covered a variety of topics about recovery and involvement in the program. Questions were designed to answer the two evaluation questions that focused on how PRS supports recovery and why it is effective. The peer conducting interviews was instructed to follow-up on responses when additional information was required, or to clarify responses provided. **Analysis-** Interview data were transcribed into Microsoft Word from handwritten and text messages sent to the evaluator. All identifying information that could be linked to informants was removed and participants received a unique identification number (#1-6). Data extraction for this evaluation involved selecting and coding all text based on interview questions. The coding structure was developed a priori (before) by the evaluator. One person coded the initial transcripts. Codes were reviewed by all authors, including those with the lived experience of recovery and involved in the program. Data analysis involved coding all of the transcripts using the a priori codes developed, then identifying key themes from the coded data. A priori themes used to code data include, the context of recovery, program impacts, spiritual aspects of recovery, and recommendations. Homelessness, fear of relapse, and the importance of social support were contextual factors that impact recovery. This is consistent with previous studies in this population where social support and housing were facilitated through peer recovery support services. Themes were reviewed by all team members to ensure they were appropriate based on context and evaluation questions. **Validation** of the results occurred by sharing the results with individuals involved in the program, and those with the lived experience of recovery, comparing results with existing literature, and consensus of results through verbal agreement of authors. **Findings-** Peers reported positive impacts from being involved in the program. Impacts related to reaching their recovery goals, achieving, and maintaining their sobriety, social connections, and community involvement. Recovery is a process and peer recovery support assists individuals by providing them with critical support when they need it most. Findings support the continued use of peer recovery support as a viable approach to maintain recovery and underscore the need for change at the individual, community, and nation levels.

Evaluation of Concurrent Disorders Group Treatment Program: Outcome Evaluation Report Example

The Canadian Mental Health Association implemented the Concurrent Disorder Project (CDP) in 2001 to address mental illness and substance use/abuse issues among clients (Aubry et al., 2003). **Intervention-** The CDP utilized group based staged treatment models (persuasion, active treatment, and relapse prevention). **Evaluation questions-** Are there changes in functioning for clients over the course of participation in the group? How do the changes in functioning over time for clients participating in the group program compared to similar clients not participating in the group program? Are there changes in the quality of life of clients over the course of participation in the group program? How do the changes in quality of life over time for clients participating in the group program compare to similar clients not participating in the group program? Does the frequency of participation in the group predict changes in functioning and quality of life of clients? **Study design-** Quasi-experimental design. The treatment group included 28 clients involved in the CDP participating in at least seven group sessions. A matched comparison group included 28 clients with concurrent disorders from CMHA without the CDP group treatment. **Data collection and analysis-** Client ratings of functioning and substance abuse were provided by clients to social workers during interviews using self-report methods. Data analyses were conducted using SPSS. Basic frequency counts and descriptive statistics were used to document the sample characteristics. To explore differences between groups authors utilized a series of repeated measures of analysis of variances (ANOVAs). **Findings-** Treatment group participants reported reductions in alcohol consumption and improved satisfaction in daily life, health, and finances. As the number of treatment sessions increased, client satisfaction levels actually decreased. A **limitation** of these findings is the small sample size, the lack of equivalent comparison group, and the short period of time under evaluation.

Meta House Recovery and Health Program Evaluation Example

The Meta House's Recovery and Health Program (R&H) is a substance abuse day treatment program for women and their families (Larson & Malcolm, 2012). With funding from SAMHSA, the R&H program target population was women with SUD, including African American women at higher risk for contracting HIV. **Goals-**The R&H goals were to improve functioning levels related to substance use and sobriety, improve mental health and self-care, reduce risk of HIV infection, and improve the family environment by promoting stability. **Evaluation questions-**To determine if these goals were met, evaluators developed the following evaluation questions: What were the characteristics of the women served by the R&H program and what were the strengths and challenges they brought with them as they entered treatment? Did women's substance use and mental health status improve after participating in the R&H program? Did women reduce their risk of HIV infection after participating in the R&H program? Were there indications of increased family stability following women's participation in the R&H program? **Evaluation design-** A non-experimental pre-post design was used. **Data collection and analysis-** Authors conducted structured interviews at entry and 1 year after the program. Interviews were based on the Government Performance Results Act (GPRA), the Addiction Severity Index (ASI), Trauma Symptom Checklist, and the Adult-Adolescent Parenting Inventory. **Findings-** R&H served 217 women, 99 completed interviews 12-months after the program started. At follow-up, 67% of women had not used alcohol or illegal drugs in the past 30-days. The R&H program decreased substance use and improved functioning overall. There were also statistically significant pre-post improvements in the number of days that women experienced mental health symptoms and in the number of different symptoms they reported. In addition, significantly fewer women were experiencing daily symptoms at follow-up (39%) as compared to intake (60%). About half of the women (50%) were not experiencing any significant mental health symptoms at 12-month follow-up. Pre-post changes in sexual risk behaviors were mixed, with a positive change in abstinence at follow-up (47%) as compared to intake (28%) (Larson & Malcolm, 2012). The 12-month follow-up data suggests that the R&H program had only limited success in meeting its goals of improving the stability of the family environment through improved parenting attitudes, increased economic self-sufficiency, and stable housing. Overall, the results show positive outcomes for women and overall, the R&H program met established goals.

ROOT Pilot Program Evaluation Example

The Recovery Opioid Overdose Team (ROOT) pilot program evaluation explored active interventions for overdose survivors in emergency departments (ED). Authors created active interventions for overdose survivors using peer recovery coaches to engage with survivors in EDs, followed by partnering with community case management navigators to connect survivors to recovery support and treatment services (Dahlem et al., 2020).

    Study design- Pilot study of ROOT intervention. The ROOT program is composed of a peer recovery coach who is in long-term recovery, and a case management navigator who specializes in mental health care and provides guidance for accessing community services. After an overdose reversal, law enforcement contacts a county 24/7 Crisis Team, who then notifies ROOT. **Intervention-**The peer recovery coach engages with the survivor in the ED, and then follow up continues with the case management navigator and the peer recovery coach for up to 90 days post-ED discharge. **Data collection and analysis-**Retrospective chart reviews were conducted to evaluate ROOT in two Midwest EDs from September 2017 through March 2019. **Findings-**Of the 122 referrals, 77.0% (n = 94) of the survivors initially engaged with ROOT in the ED or in the community. The remaining 23.0% (n = 28) left the ED against medical advice or were unengaged. The majority of overdose survivors were male (63.9%; n = 78), White (43.4%; n = 53), had housing (80.2%; n = 48), and access to transportation (48.4%; n = 59). From the 122 referrals, 33.6% (n = 41) received ongoing treatment services (n = 20 outpatient, n = 17 residential, n = 2 detoxification facility, n = 1 recovery housing, n = 1 medication treatment for opioid use disorder), 2.5% (n = 3) were incarcerated, 2.5% (n = 3) died, and 61.5% (n = 75) declined services. The ROOT, a community-wide coordinated program in the EDs, shows promise in linking overdose survivors to recovery support and treatment services post-overdose (Dahlem et al., 2020).

Outcome Evaluation of Forever Free Substance Abuse Treatment Program

The Forever Free Program started in 1991 at the California Institution for Women in Frontera. Women are being placed in the criminal justice system at higher rates than men, they have different treatment needs than men, yet most treatment programs do not have services specifically for women. The lack of services leads to relapse of drug use and high rates of recidivism. Forever Free is an intensive residential program for women inmates with substance abuse problems providing in-person treatment, in-person services, access to consulting, educational workshops, transition, and aftercare supports. Forever Free aimed to reduce the number of disciplinary actions women experienced in prison, seduce substance abuse, and reduce recidivism (Pendergast, 2003). **Study design-** Evaluators created a non-randomized quasi experimental design with comparison group. The treatment **sampling frame** included all clients entering the program from 1997 to 1998 of these 119 agreed to participate. The comparison sample included women attending the Life Plan for Recovery eight-week education session. The comparison sampling frame included all clients that enrolled in the course from April to November 1998, of these 96 agreed to participate. **Data collection-** Background information and standardized instruments that measure drug and alcohol use, relationships, treatment, social support, psychological status, vocational training, and criminal activity were collected at follow-up. Baseline data were collected at the beginning of the intervention from treatment and comparison groups. Follow-up data collection occurred 1 year after clients were released from prison, 84% of the participants were reached. **Data analysis-** All data were analyzed using SAS and SPSS chi-square and t-test procedures. **Findings-** Forever Free participants reported fewer arrests, convictions, or incarcerations since release from prison. At 6 months post-release, 40% of the comparison group were incarcerated compared to just 15% of the treatment group. Other favorable outcomes reported by the treatment group include decreased drug use, increased employment, improved treatment motivation, improved relationships with children and more participants reunited with their children. **Recommendations** from this evaluation call for mandated community aftercare, service needs assessment prior to parole, linking participants to community services, vocational training, more research on cognitive-behavioral health treatment in prison, and additional research on post-release services on desired long-term outcomes (Pendergast, 2003).

Wrap Up

Evaluating treatment programs is not a straightforward process. A public health approach to treatment program evaluation requires evaluators to use the best available data and make decisions that consider the seven future generations. Examples of various evaluation products, from the needs assessment and program development process to the implementation of the evaluation, including quantitative and qualitative data collection and analysis serve as a guide for evaluators wanting to know how to make sense of all of the data we collect. This chapter also reviewed common treatment program variables such as those from NOMs, and GPRA intake and follow-up data requirements. There are many paths to recovery and many paths to evaluating treatment programs. Remember that whatever path that you choose, you will encounter difficulty. Stay focused on a public health approach, equity, and justice. What determines health? How do we know? Evaluation.

Discussion Questions

1. What are the principles that guide all evaluators mentioned earlier in this chapter?
2. What are NOMs data and how might they be used in an evaluation?
3. Describe the application of the SDOH in a treatment program evaluation? What questions do you still have about SDOH focused evaluation?
4. Discuss the evaluation examples presented, the types of evaluation designs, data collection approaches, analysis methods, and findings.

Additional Resources

Bureau of Justice Assistance Prescription Drug Monitoring Program (PDMP), http://www.namsdl.org/prescription-monitoring-programs.cfm

Centers for Disease Control Behavioral Risk Factor Surveillance System (BRFSS), https://www.cdc.gov/brfss/index.html

Centers for Disease Control and Prevention National Syndromic Surveillance Program,

https://www.cdc.gov/nssp/index.html

Centers for Disease Control WONDER,

https://wonder.cdc.gov/

Centers for Disease Control Youth Risk Behavior Surveillance System (YRBSS), https://www.cdc.gov/healthyyouth/data/yrbs/index.htm

Center for Substance Abuse Treatment. Substance Abuse Treatment for Persons

With Co-Occurring Disorders. Screening and Assessment Instruments, https://www.ncbi.nlm.nih.gov/books/NBK64190/?report=classic

Drug Abuse Treatment Cost Analysis Program, http://www.datcap.com/

Federal Bureau of Investigation Uniform Crime Reporting Program, https://www.fbi.gov/services/cjis/ucr

Medicare Part D Prescriber Data, Centers for Medicare and Medicaid Services, https://www.cms.gov/research-statistics-data-and-systems/statistics-trends-and-reports/medicare-provider-charge-data/part-d-prescriber.html

National Survey on Drug Use and Health (NSDUH), https://nsduhweb.rti.org/respweb/homepage.cfm

Substance Abuse and Mental Health Services Administration NOMs Client-Level Measures Guide for Adults, https://spars.samhsa.gov/sites/default/files/CMHSAdultClientLvlSvcsMeasQxQ_3.17.2020.pdf

US Department of Justice Automation of Reports and Consolidated Orders System (ARCOS), https://www.deadiversion.usdoj.gov/arcos/index.html

US Department of Veterans Affairs https://www.hsrd.research.va.gov/research/portfolio_description.cfm?Sulu=32

References

American Evaluation Association. (2018). *Guiding principles for evaluators.* https://www.eval.org/About/Guiding-Principles

Aubry, T., Cousins, B., LaFerriere, D., & Wexler, A. (2003). *Evaluation of concurrent disorders group treatment program: outcome evaluation report.* Centre for Research on Community Services Faculty of Social Sciences, University of Ottawa. https://www.evaluationcanada.ca/distribution/200308_aubry_tim_cousins_brad_laferriere_diane_wexler_audrey.pdf

Baker, T. E., & Chang, G. (2016). The use of auricular acupuncture in opioid use disorder: A systematic literature review. *The American Journal on Addictions, 25*(8), 592–602. 10.1111/ajad.12453

Bronfenbrenner, U. (1979). *The ecology of human development: Experiments by nature and design.* Harvard University Press.

Bryman, A., & Burgess, B. (Eds.). (1994). *Analyzing qualitative data.* Routledge. 10.4324/9780203413081

Chaudhury, R., Jones, H. E., Wechsberg, W., O'Grady, K. E., Tuten, M., & Chisolm, M. S. (2010). Addiction severity index composite scores as predictors for sexual-risk behaviors and drug-use behaviors in drug-using pregnant patients. *The American Journal of Drug and Alcohol Abuse, 36*(1), 25–30. 10.3109/00952990903544810

Coughlin, S. S., Mann, P., Vernon, M., Young, L., Ayyala, D., Sams, R., & Hatzigeorgiou, C. (2019). A logic framework for evaluating social determinants of health interventions in primary care. *Journal of Hospital Management and Health Policy, 3*, 23. 10.21037/jhmhp.2019.09.03

Dahlem, C. H. (Gina), Scalera, M., Anderson, G., Tasker, M., Ploutz-Snyder, R., McCabe, S. E., & Boyd, C. J. (2020). Recovery opioid overdose team (ROOT) pilot program evaluation: A community-wide post-overdose response strategy. *Substance Abuse, 0*(0), 1–5. 10.1080/08897077.2020.1847239

De Ver Dye, T., Muir, E., Farovitch, L., Siddiqi, S., & Sharma, S. (2020). Critical medical ecology and SARS-COV-2 in the urban environment: A pragmatic, dynamic approach to explaining and planning for research and practice. *Infectious Diseases of Poverty*, 9(1), 71. 10.1186/s40249-020-00694-3

Ettner, S. L., Huang, D., Evans, E., Rose Ash, D., Hardy, M., Jourabchi, M., & Hser, Y.-I. (2006). Benefit–cost in the California treatment outcome project: Does substance abuse treatment "pay for itself"? *Health Services Research*, 41(1), 192–213. 10.1111/j.1475-6773.2005.00466.x

Fisher, P. A., & Ball, T. J. (2003). Tribal Participatory Research: Mechanisms of a Collaborative Model. *American Journal of Community Psychology*, 32(3-4), 207–216. https://doi-org.libproxy.uncg.edu/10.1023/b:ajcp.0000004742.39858.c5

Kelley, A., Bingham, D., Brown, E., & Pepion, L. (2017). Assessing the impact of American Indian peer recovery support on substance use and health. *Journal of Groups in Addiction & Recovery*, 12(4), 296–308. 10.1080/1556035X.2017.1337531

Kelley, A., McCoy, T., Fisher, A., Witzel, M., Fatupaito, B., & Restad, D. (2020). Comparability of survey measures in hard to reach populations: Methods and recommendations. *Practical Assessment Research and Evaluation*. 25(9), 13.

Kelley, A., Piccione, C., Fisher, A., Matt, K., Andreini, M., & Bingham, D. (2019). Survey development: Community involvement in the design and implementation process. *Journal of Public Health Management and Practice: JPHMP, 25 Suppl 5, Tribal Epidemiology Centers: Advancing Public Health in Indian Country for Over 20 Years*, S77–S83. 10.1097/PHH.0000000000001016

Kelley, A., Steinberg, R., McCoy, T. P., Pack, R., & Pepion, L. (2021). Exploring recovery: Findings from a six-year evaluation of an American Indian peer recovery support program. *Drug and Alcohol Dependence*, 221, 108559. 10.1016/j.drugalcdep.2021.108559

Kelley, A., Witzel, M., & Fatupaito, B. (2019). Preventing substance use in American Indian youth: The case for social support and community connections. *Substance Use & Misuse*, 54(5), 787–795. 10.1080/10826084.2018.1536724

Kelly, P. J., Kyngdon, F., Ingram, I., Deane, F. P., Baker, A. L., & Osborne, B. A. (2018). The client satisfaction questionnaire-8: Psychometric properties in a cross-sectional survey of people attending residential substance abuse treatment. *Drug and Alcohol Review*, 37(1), 79–86. 10.1111/dar.12522

Kunins, H. V., Sohler, N. L., Giovanniello, A., Thompson, D., & Cunningham, C. O. (2013). A buprenorphine education and training program for primary care residents: Implementation and evaluation. *Substance Abuse: Official Publication of the Association for Medical Education and Research in Substance Abuse*, 34(3), 242–247. 10.1080/08897077.2012.752777

Larson, L., & Malcolm, E. (2012). *Final program evaluation report for meta houses's recovery and health program*. Planning Council for Health and Humans Services, Inc. https://www.impactinc.org/fileadmin/user_upload/planning-council/pdfs/RH-Evaluation-Final-Report-FINAL.pdf

Lee, S., & Jo, D.-H. (2019). Acupuncture for reduction of opioid consumption in chronic pain. *Medicine*, 98(51), e18237. 10.1097/MD.0000000000018237

McLeroy, K. R., Bibeau, D., Steckler, A., & Glanz, K. (1988). An ecological perspective on health promotion programs. *Health Education Quarterly*, 15(4), 351–377. 10.1177/109019818801500401

Palinkas, L. A., Horwitz, S. M., Green, C. A., Wisdom, J. P., Duan, N., & Hoagwood, K. (2015). Purposeful sampling for qualitative data collection and analysis in mixed method implementation research. *Administration and Policy in Mental Health*, 42(5), 533–544. 10.1007/s10488-013-0528-y

Pendergast, M. (2003). *Outcome evaluation of the forever free substance abuse treatment program: one-year post-release outcomes.* National Institute of Justice. https://www.ojp.gov/ncjrs/virtual-library/abstracts/outcome-evaluation-forever-free-substance-abuse-treatment-program

Pinto, A. D., Glattstein-Young, G., Mohamed, A., Bloch, G., Leung, F.-H., & Glazier, R. H. (2016). Building a foundation to reduce health inequities: Routine collection of sociodemographic data in primary care. *The Journal of the American Board of Family Medicine*, 29(3), 348–355. 10.3122/jabfm.2016.03.150280

Recovery Centers of America. (n.d.). Economic cost of substance abuse in the United States, 2016. *Recovery Centers of America.* Retrieved September 10, 2021, from https://recoverycentersofamerica.com/economic-cost-substance-abuse/

Rogers, J. L., Gilbride, D. D., & Dew, B. J. (2018). Utilizing an ecological framework to enhance counselors' understanding of the U.S. opioid epidemic. *The Professional Counselor*, 8(3), 226–239. 10.15241/jlr.8.3.226

Rural Health Information Hub. (n.d.). *Evaluation tools – RHIhub mental health toolkit.* Retrieved July 16, 2021, from https://www.ruralhealthinfo.org/toolkits/mental-health/5/evaluation-tools

SAMHSA. (n.d.). *Grants.* Retrieved October 22, 2021, from https://www.samhsa.gov/grants

SAMHSA. (2019). *CMHS national outcome measures (NOMs) client-level measures for discretionary programs providing direct services question-by-question instruction guide for adult programs.* 78. https://spars.samhsa.gov/sites/default/files/CMHSAdultClientLvlSvcsMeasQxQ_3.17.2020.pdf

Thomas, G. (2005). *Addiction Treatment Indicators in Canada: An Environmental Scan.* Ottawa, ON: Canadian Centre on Substance Abuse. National Policy Working Group Policy Discussion Document. https://www.researchgate.net/profile/Gerald-Thomas/publication/237525602_Addiction_Treatment_Indicators_in_Canada_An_Environmental_Scan/links/0046353399c3d3f746000000/Addiction-Treatment-Indicators-in-Canada-An-Environmental-Scan.pdf

6 The Public Health Approach to Treatment and Recovery

CONTENTS

DOI: 10.4324/9781003290728-6

Learning Objectives

After reading this chapter, you should be able to:

- Apply the public health approach to treatment program evaluation to multiple treatments and recovery models.
- Discuss the impacts of COVID-19 on treatment, access, and recovery.
- Distinguish between small "p" and big "P" policies and how they relate to treatment program context and recovery.
- Provide examples of policies, systems, and environmental change and discuss how they support a public health approach to treatment and recovery.

A Public Health Approach

Throughout this text, we have reviewed different approaches to treatment and recovery. Approaches are mixed in their effectiveness; evaluation of these approaches varies from a descriptive evaluation to a full-blown quasi-experimental evaluation. A fundamental difference in a public health approach to treatment is that it continually seeks to understand problems, causes, solutions, and support the widespread adoption of effective treatment programs. Not for the weak at heart or easily discouraged, the public health approach is relentless and requires a systematic way of defining problems and finding solutions (Figure 6.1).

In this chapter, we will zero-in on public health approaches and frameworks. Values of health equity and social justice will guide us as we will explore determinants, conditions, policies, and structures that impact treatment and health program effectiveness and our ability to be effective as evaluators. Public health can be radical. Wicked problems require out-of-the-box, innovative, and creative solutions. As advocates of a public health approach, I give us (you and me) permission to be radical.

Public Health Approach to Evaluating Substance Misuse Treatment Programs

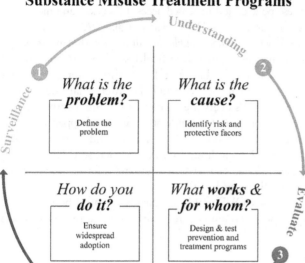

Figure 6.1 Public Health Approach to Substance Misuse Treatment.

COVID-19 Impacts

You probably know about the COVID-19 pandemic we have been enduring for nearly 2 years. COVID-19 has consumed public health workers, evaluators, educators, researchers, and providers. We have all lost something, friends and colleagues to the disease, time with our loved ones, in-person classes, and missed preventative medical screening appointments. COVID-19 uncovered some wicked problems with power, misinformation, and disinformation in mass media, and the impact it has on what we believe, and how we act. Glaring disparities in health infrastructure, policies, and systems that support health became very clear. With rich countries hoarding the vaccine and Low to Middle Income Countries (LMICs) not having enough of the vaccine for their most vulnerable populations in need.

But the impacts of COVID-19 are not all bad. Policies around OUD, telehealth, and medication-assisted treatment (MAT) are less restrictive because of COVID-19. Insurance now reimburses for psychotherapy and other health services delivered via virtual conferencing or telephone—this is new, thank you COVID and policymakers. SAMSHA recently lifted regulations on methadone dispensing practices, before COVID-19 individuals were required to access a methadone clinic daily (yes daily) for their prescription. Now, individuals can now take home a 14–28 day supply of methadone (Bao et al., 2020). Social and recreational recovery infrastructure and social media have increased as well, with more than 10,000 apps to address mental health alone (Henry et al., 2020). Yet, experts call for more research and evaluation to explore the impacts of these policies and increased access to services and medication resulting from policy change during COVID-19 (Henry et al., 2020).

In a practical sense, COVID-19 made *public health* a term that most people know and appreciate. Terms we use in public health such as prevention, surveillance, disease, infection rates, morbidity and mortality, intervention, and policy are more known. I asked my 12-year-old daughter what she thought public health meant, she said, "It's everyone … people coming together to help out, prevent diseases, care for one another, understand what is happening." How has COVID-19 impacted you? How do you, your family, and your community view public health? As a term? As a discipline? As an approach? I believe the COVID-19 pandemic has opened our eyes to human suffering and the importance of community in all things health.

Public Health Takeaway—COVID-19 has radically changed how we think about public health and how we communicate health information to the world.

Institute of Medicine

The Institute of Medicine (IOM) created a public health prevention framework that includes two existing prevention models. This framework advocates for addressing health inequities, structural inequities, and the social determinants of health (SDOH). Within their new model, IOM intervention classifications are presented including universal, selective, and indicated programs and interventions. Now, I cannot believe this is a public health evaluation textbook and we are just getting to this figure (Figure 6.2) but bear with me. This IOM approach targets individuals based on their level of risk where **universal strategies** include

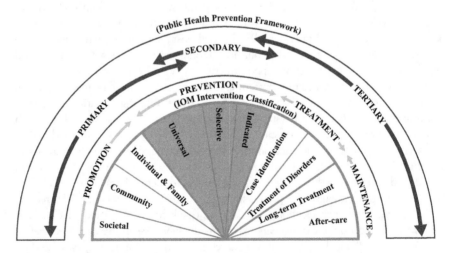

Figure 6.2 Institute of Medicine Public Health Prevention Framework. (Source: Adapted from NASEM, 2020).

an entire population, **selective strategies** target a subset of the population that may be placed at greater risk and experience greater inequities, **indicated strategies** are designed for a select group of a population that has an undesirable health outcome, such as addiction (National Academies of Science, Engineering, and Medicine [NASEM], 2020).

NASEM writes, "**Health inequities**" are systematic differences in opportunities that lead to unfair and avoidable differences in health (p. 18). **Structural inequities** are the result of unequal distribution of power and resources based on race, gender, class, sexual orientation, gender expression, and or other identities (p.18). Understanding these terms and using the IOM prevention framework (and others) may help evaluators as they develop equity-focused evaluations.

A public health approach **calls for action** that addresses health inequities and structural inequities (for everyone, all places, people, ages, genders, races/ethnicities, and status). Another useful model is the **disease model of public health**. You may be familiar with this from the COVID-19 pandemic, it is often presented using an agent, host, and environment model, where the threats to public health are based on the 1) host (person susceptible), 2) infectious agent, and 3) environment. Experts have used this model in MHSU domains, to illustrate prevention strategies, skill-building, intervention targets, and exposures. Harm reduction is one clear example of the disease model of public health. Harm reduction approaches include designated drivers, drug consumption rooms, or syringe needle exchange programs (SNEPS). These approaches aim to lessen the public health impacts of MHSU and addiction by providing alternatives that overall reduce harm.

Rat Parks and Models of Addiction

Recall the various models we reviewed in Chapter 2 about addiction (Alexander et al., 1978). The **Rat Park** experiments tell us that the social environment drives addiction or sobriety (Gage & Sumnall, 2019). In contrast, the disease model of addiction is a **causal model**, where the brain is defected by drugs or alcohol, and disease symptoms result from consumption (Pickard, 2017). The **socioecological model** was also discussed as a way to examine public health issues such as addiction that have a behavioral health component. By looking at causal relationships and feedback loops (remember general systems theory), we can begin to understand what is happening at the environmental, community, and social levels. Although in direct contrast to the disease model of addiction, we also reviewed the **learning model of addiction**, where addiction is viewed as the product of learning and development which can be overcome by more learning, development, empowerment, and some would say self-*actualization* (Lewis, 2017).

Radical Public Health

Public health requires us to step out of what we think we know … . We defend our favorite theories and models at the podium, and we preach about our research until we can no longer speak, or nobody will listen. We publish papers and posters with the crazy idea that we will change minds. But we do not. Being a radical public health evaluator, professional, researcher, and leader (whatever you are, and we are), we have to put aside the podium failures and the inability to convert die-hard theorists to another way of thinking about addiction. We have to come together as one strong and impermeable unit, committed to the relentless pursuit of public health, health equity, and social justice. Who is with me? How about the radical idea of decriminalizing addiction?

Drug addiction is a complex public health problem that is preventable and treatable. The 2016 United Nations General Assembly Special Session (UNGASS) on drugs met to discuss scientific evidence for the concept that SUDs are brain disorders and that people recover when they have access to evidence-based treatment and social support (Volkow et al., 2017). UNGASS echoed what other evaluators, researchers, and policymakers know, criminal justice, and punitive approaches to addressing SUD are not effective, and they do more harm than good (Chandler et al., 2009).

Decriminalizing Addiction

Despite gains in scientific knowledge and mounting evidence that addiction is a brain disease, individuals with addiction are more likely to be incarcerated because of their disease. Advocates, researchers, and policymakers call for decriminalizing addiction as one path forward. This work is happening throughout the United States, Volkow, the leader at NIDA calls for a public health approach to addressing SUD rather than criminalizing it (Volkow, 2021). This approach calls for multiple stakeholders and systems to come forward (law enforcement, courts, health care providers and systems, insurance companies, and recovery-oriented systems of care). One of the goals of decriminalizing addiction is to build racial equity and to ensure that individuals from racial and ethnic minority groups receive fair, equitable, and effective treatment (and support). Volkow points to several inequities in the current US systems that must change. First, there is **no equitable enforcement**. White and Black people report similar rates of drug use, yet Black people are four times more likely to be arrested for drug possession than Whites (Volkow, 2021). Moreover, 56% of the people in prison for a drug offense are either African American or Latino but combined these populations only make up 25% of the US population. Second, current **punishment approaches are ineffective**. Imprisonment for drugs and other offenses leads to a higher risk of drug overdose when inmates are released. At least half of the people in prison have an untreated SUD and an estimated 65% of the US prison population has an SUD (National Institute on Drug Abuse, 2020). Third, **inequitable access to treatment** has been documented in numerous studies. One study reports that it took Black people 4–5 years longer to access additional treatment than Whites. Minority groups in the United States are less likely to receive MAT than White patients (Volkow, 2020). Fourth, **the vicious cycle of punishment for addiction must end** because it is not working. A recent report by the Pew Charitable Trust reports that more lengthy prison terms do not reduce drug use, distribution, or other drug-law violations (Pew Charitable Trust, 2018). A public health approach to decriminalizing addiction requires effective policies at multiple levels, these include law enforcement strategies, alternative sentencing strategies, treatment strategies, and prevention strategies. Can you imagine if the United States started criminalizing type 2 diabetes? How many people would we have in our prison systems? **The Human Rights Watch Report** reminds us that every 25 seconds in the United States someone is incarcerated because of drug possession for their personal use (Borden, 2016). Policies that criminalize drugs are a public health failure and an example of one of the many policies that must change.

Harm Reduction

The AIDS epidemic in the 1980s elevated harm reduction models as a public health solution to reducing HIV infection by providing syringe and needle exchange programs (SNEPS) for persons who inject drugs (PWID). As a public health alternative to the moral and criminal models of drug use and addiction, harm reduction models advocate for integrative and holistic responses to address drug use and other high-risk behaviors. Harm reduction approaches discussed in Marlatt's seminal article, Harm Reduction: Come as You Are (1996) propelled a revolution in the United States and challenged policymakers to think beyond the moral model and war on drugs and the disease model of addiction (Marlatt, 1996). Marlatt (and others) advocate the harm reduction approach, "Harm reduction normalizes these high-risk behaviors by placing them in the context of acquired habits, learned behaviors that are strengthened by the influence of powerful reinforcers. Harm reduction defines much drug use, and perhaps certain high-risk sexual activities as well, as maladaptive coping responses rather than as indicators of either physical illness or personal immorality" (Marlatt, 1996, p. 787).

Principles

In the last 40 years, progress in harm reduction models is evident and the National Council on Harm Reduction established the following principles for harm reduction practice: 1) accepts for better or worse that drug use is part of the world and works to minimize its effect rather than ignore or condemn, 2) understands that drug use is a complex and multi-faceted issue that includes a spectrum of behaviors from sever use to abstinence and acknowledges that some drugs use practices are safer than others, 3) establishes the quality of individual and community life and wellbeing as the criteria for successful interventions and policies (opposed to abstinence), 4) calls for non-judgmental, non-coercive provision of services and resources for people who use drugs and the communities where they live to assist them with reducing possible harm (Harm Reduction Coalition, n.d.). Indeed, harm reduction is a pragmatic approach that advocates for human rights of people who use drugs (Des Jarlais, 2017) and supports a decriminalization stance.

Public Health Takeaway- The message *come as you are* is one message that every public health program, treatment center, community initiative must embrace for real change to happen.

The **Community Care in Reach** mobile health initiative promotes harm education and medication for OUD for high-risk populations. The Kraft Center for Community at Massachusetts General Hospital partnered with Boston Health Care for the Homeless Program (BHCHP) and the Boston Public Health Commission (BPHC) to launch an innovative mobile health initiative targeting opioid overdose "hotspots" in Greater Boston. With an impressive mobile white and blue van, the initiative provides various program services (MAT, detox-ification, pre- and post-exposure prophylaxis for HIV, referrals to behavioral therapy), primary care services (screenings, vaccinations, wound care, tele-behavioral health consults, and referrals for specialty care), and harm reduction services (syringe exchange and collection, naloxone distribution and training, counseling on reducing risk when using drugs, and drug residue testing) (Regis et al., 2020). Regis and colleagues utilized a mixed-method evaluation approach to evaluate the Community Care in Reach pilot program. **Findings show significant impacts**, reaching 3,800 people who use drugs and 308 clinical encounters during the first 10 months of programming. The mobile care approach increased access to buprenorphine treatment and demonstrates it is possible to deliver buprenorphine in a mobile setting with 47 patients receiving treatment. Another central finding from the evaluation was that more than half of the patients served by the mobile care approach were new to the BHCHP services, demonstrating that a mobile approach has the potential to reach new patients and increase access and utilization to other services (treatment, social services, preventive, and more). Qualitative data collected from patients underscore the benefits of this approach with patients reporting positive experiences, compassionate and helpful staff. Authors report, "Too many individuals never make it through the doors of our brick-and-mortar institutions to access the addiction care and services they need" (Regis et al., 2020, p. 7).

Drug Courts

Drug courts reduce recidivism rates for individuals with substance-related offenses and many advocates view drug courts as a public health approach and solution to the criminalization of drugs. Developed in the 1990s for non-violent offenders, drug courts generally include multidisciplinary teams including judges, prosecutors, social workers, corrections officials, attorneys, and treatment program staff. Family and community are encouraged to participate in hearings and drug court programs, including graduation from drug courts.

Gibbs and colleagues conducted a study of 824 drug court participants to determine the effects of criminal sentencing on recidivism. They explored the association between recidivism and case dismissal, probation, jail, and prison over 1–3 year follow-up periods. **Their results show** that 15% of participants offended within the first year in the community after completing the drug court program, 29% reoffended after 2 years, and 37% offended after 3 years (Gibbs et al., 2019). Recidivism was more common in participants who did not graduate from drug courts. Researchers also found that imprisonment did not deter or prevent recidivism in drug court failures. They recommend sentencing drug court failures to community-based alternatives as opposed to a fixed period of incarceration.

Trauma and Addiction: A Public Health Approach

Trauma refers to events that involve actual or threatened risk of death, serious injury, or sexual violation. Most people will experience at least one traumatic event in their lifetimes but sometimes more (Substance Abuse and Mental Health Services Administration, 2018). Trauma and addiction are relatives, they show up together, or not far behind. **SAMHSA reports that 92% of homeless women with children have severe trauma histories** and twice the rate of drug and alcohol dependence compared with women without trauma histories (Substance Abuse and Mental Health Services Administration, 2011). Veterans seek treatment for SUD and PTSD, with nearly one-third of veterans reporting both (Substance Abuse and Mental Health Services Administration, 2018). Researchers have studied trauma extensively and developed public health models for preventing trauma at the individual, family, community, and national levels. Yet equity is still missing in the trauma milieu where age, gender, race/ethnicity, and sexual orientation predict who will experience trauma and how much they will experience. Trauma during childhood, Adverse Childhood Experiences (ACEs), impact cognitive development, social and emotional functioning, and lead to the adoption of health risk behaviors that may increase MHSUD. Efforts to address trauma and prevent ACES are widespread. Here are some examples:

The **International Society for Traumatic Stress Studies (ISTSS)** developed a report, A Public Health Approach to Trauma: Implications for Science, Practice, Policy, and the Role of the ISTSS (International Society for Traumatic Stress Studies, 2015). This comprehensive report outlines the public health impacts of trauma, a public health model of traumatic stress, and the importance of public health policies in addressing trauma. Authors promote the socioecological model as a framework for the prevention of trauma, observing the individual, relationship, community, and societal levels as points for intervention and prevention. Targets of preventive interventions are conceptualized through a linear model where primary, secondary, and tertiary approaches are used to intervene, at various time points from exposure, disorder, and outcomes.

Another approach is the **Community Resilience Model.** Developed by the Trauma Resource Institute, individuals and communities learn how to build trauma-informed resilience-focused throughout the world. CRM and the Trauma Resilience Model (TRM) are based on the biology of traumatic stress reactions and teaching individual skills to return the mind, body, and spirit after traumatic events (Grabbe & Miller-Karas, 2017).

Bethel and colleagues synthesized theoretical and empirical evidence about ACEs, resilience, and fostering healthy development across the lifespan. Their research resulted in the following priorities for policy and agenda setting: 1) translation of ACES, resilience, and relationships, 2) cultivate conditions to address structural inequalities, restore and reward safe and nurturing relationships, and support launch and learn efforts to address ACEs (Bethell et al., 2017).

Community-Based Strategies

Researchers at the University of Kansas and the World Health Organization conceptualized *Seven Strategies for Community Change.* An approach that combines individual and environmental strategies to create a comprehensive framework that includes everyone in the community. Seven strategies for community change are as follows:

1. Provide information—individual level
2. Build skills—individual level
3. Provide support—individual level
4. Enhance access and reduce barriers—community level
5. Change consequences and incentives—community level
6. Change physical design of the environment—community level
7. Change rules and policy—community level (CADCA, 2018)

Ohio implemented a community-driven, collective impact approach to address the growing opioid crisis and focused on the social determinants of health (SDOH). Ohio's model, the Community Collective Impact Model for Change initiative was implemented over a 2-year period reaching 18 communities across the state. A key focus of Ohio's work was addressing trauma. They reached 18 communities and increased multi-sector collaborations, implemented strategies to mobilize communities around trauma, and developed community-level strategic plans for prevention, treatment, and recovery (Raffle & Leach, 2020).

A Community-Based Public Health Approach to Suicide Prevention

I evaluated a series of SAMSHA-funded suicide prevention programs for 10 years in one rural tribal community. **Goals of this evaluation** were to support a public health approach to suicide prevention by collecting community data and developing prevention approaches based on needs identified in the data. In this community, there was not a standard definition of suicide, so the first step was to define suicide based on cultural and historical definitions (Kelley et al., 2015). For example, some community members viewed suicide as a spirit that comes to help those in spiritual pain and also a spiritual guide that comes to listen and guide individuals in need of help. Others defined it using biomedical terms, considering it as an individual's thoughts or actions that may include ideation, attempt, or physical death caused by self-directed injurious behavior. We considered both definitions and developed a survey to document risk and protective factors of youth in the community. **Using a CBPR approach** and tenets of the inter-personal theory of suicide as a guide, we explored social support, depression, self-esteem, anxiety, stress, and suicide ideation. The community collected more than 100 surveys from youth, the strongest correlations were correlations among variables were depression and suicide ideation ($r = .711$, $p < .01$), depression and stressful life events ($r = .580$, $p < .01$), antisocial behaviors and suicide ideation ($r = .505$, $p < .01$), and anxiety and stressful life events ($r = .520$, $p < .01$). As expected, self-esteem scores were negatively correlated with SIQ scores, depression, antisocial behaviors, and social support. Females were more likely to report significantly higher mean scores for all psychosocial risk factors with the exception of the protective factor, self-esteem, where males reported significantly higher levels of self-esteem. As age increased, anxiety, depression, and suicide ideation increased, whereas antisocial behaviors decreased. **Results** demonstrated that depression scores were associated with suicide ideation. While depression was the strongest independent risk factor for suicide ideation in this evaluation, the etiology of depression among youth in this community is different. Underlying factors and environmental conditions such as poverty, racism, discrimination, poor quality education, poor housing, limited access to healthcare, and limited social supports place these youth at higher risk for suicide. Thinking back on this evaluation, our efforts increased the community's understanding about suicide, and identified factors and conditions that contribute to increased risk, morbidity, and morality. The public health approach was effective in documenting the problem, and even understanding causes (steps 1–2), but we failed to determine if the prevention and early intervention approaches that we implemented were effective in reducing risk factors and suicides in the community (Kelley et al., 2018).

Public Health Takeaway- A public health approach to treatment program evaluation requires that we consider policies, systems, and environmental change that is necessary for change. A key focus on public health approaches is their use of policies that impact populations as opposed to practices that impact individuals. The next section explores this in greater detail.

Policies that Fail to Support a Public Health Approach

I do not want to sound pessimistic, but our public health policies have failed us. A 2012 **Institute of Medicine** (IOM) Report, For the Public's Health:

Investing in a Healthier Future, called attention to serious public health system deficiencies and the need for comprehensive policies and practices that support the integration of care into population health (Institute of Medicine, 2012). IOM called for adequate and sustainable funding, reform of public health infrastructure, funding, and operations based on need, and using public health knowledge and evidence to improve quality and delivery of care reaching populations. The IOM report and overall recommendations fail to address addiction as a public health problem, and brain disease.

Alegría and colleagues summarized policy goals for mental health and addiction services in their 2021 publication. They targeted existing policies, responsible parties, and actions that need to occur for equity and innovation, and public health (Alegría et al., 2021) (Table 6.1).

Table 6.1 Policies that Fail Public Health and Recommended Actions for Policy Change

Big "P" Policies	Responsible Party	Recommended Actions for Public Health
Mainstream Addiction Treatment Act (H.R.2482) (Tonko, 2019a)	Drug Enforcement Agency (DEA)	End waiver requirements for physicians to prescribe buprenorphine for addiction treatment.
Reduce Barriers to SU Treatment Act (H.R.3925) (Tonko, 2019b)	Medicaid	End-state restrictions on federal Medicaid funding for MAT/SUD
Health Insurance Portability and Accountability Act (HIPPA) 1996	Health Resources and Services Administration (HRSA) and Health and Human Services (HHS)	Permanent changes to COVID-19 policies that expand telehealth services, providers, and locations
Crisis Care Improvement and Suicide Prevention Act of 2020	SAMHSA	Block grant funding to create crisis response systems in every state
Medicaid Re-entry Act (H.R.1329) (Brownley, 2021)	Medicaid	Medicaid pays for coverage of individuals 30 days before they are released from jail/prisons, integrated re-entry system
Health Equity and Accountability Act of 2020 (H.R. 6637) (Garcia, 2020)	HRSA	Create programs for minority populations, address social determinants, mental health disorders, rural areas, Indian Health Service, mental health research in schools, and at the border

Adapted from Alegría et al., 2021.

There are other examples of Policies that fail to support a public health approach to treatment and recovery. The **Americans with Disabilities Act** (ADA) does not allow employers to treat employees or potential employees differently because of their disabilities. However, ADA does not recognize current illegal drug use as a disability. Employers may fire, demote, or terminate employees who seek treatment for addiction (Americans with Disabilities Act, ND). Another big "P" law that impacts individuals with SUD is the **Fair Housing Laws** (HUD, ND). This Law allows landlords and federal subsidized housing agencies to deny individuals housing because of illegal drug use. Advocates **of 42 CFR Part 2 (HIPPA)** call for greater confidentiality. Currently, HIPPA allows healthcare providers to share information about patient SUD with law enforcement, judges, and others who may subpoena the information. Unfortunately, there is no requirement of confidentiality during legal proceedings. Sharing information about a patient's SUD status may perpetuate stigma, discrimination, and treatment bias in the healthcare system.

Unmet Public Health Policy Needs

There are countless public health policy failures and opportunities. Consider that just 8% of medical schools in the United States require students to complete a course on addiction medicine (SAMHSA & Office of the Surgeon General, 2017). Public health professionals working in a variety of disciplines from educators to pharmacists or infectious disease specialists are not required to complete any courses or education about SUD. Policies are needed that require medical students and public health professionals to complete professional courses in SUD. This glaring gap in educational requirements of medical providers and public health policy leaders may contribute to the lack of understanding that addiction is preventable and treatable. In addition, integrating treatment for MHSUD into general healthcare settings is needed but lacking. New policies that screen individuals at risk for SUD could go a long way in preventing and treating addiction as a disease.

Policy, Systems, and Environmental Change for the Prevention and Treatment of SUD

The prevention and treatment of SUD require a multi-pronged public health approach. Another model used to explore overlapping strategies is the policy, systems, and environmental change (PSE) framework. PSE focuses on specific aspects of change required for effective treatment. Let's consider some key terms. A **public health policy** may be a law, regulation, action, decision, or practice that promotes wellness and health. Public health policies informed by evidence can prevent and treat SUD. **Systems change** is a mindset or an approach to solving problems based on an organization or institution's culture, policies, practices, and beliefs. **Environmental change** may include economic, social, physical, or cultural conditions that contribute to SUD. Environmental change strategies are most effective when combined with other strategies. The next section presents policy examples related to the prevention, treatment, and recovery for individuals and communities.

Policies

Public Health Policies and Approaches

The development of public health policies (state, local, federal, grassroots) to address SUD are essential in promoting health equity, preventing the onset of disease, and providing effective treatment. But public health policy change is difficult, it takes time, and it is not for those who give up easily. One distinction in thinking about policies is how public health policy systems vary in how they utilize evidence at the local, state, or federal level. Policies can be viewed as big "P" policies or small "p" *policies*. Big "P" policies include formal laws, rules, and regulations enacted by local In contrast small "p" policies are those that come from organizations, agency decisions, social norms, or agreements (Brownson et al., 2009). Let's consider some big "P" policies and small "p" policies in public health. The most well-established big "P" public health policy informed by scientific evidence is the 1964 Surgeon General's Report on Smoking and Health. The acknowledgment of the deleterious effects of tobacco was not federally recognized for years despite convincing evidence from epidemiologists, animal experiments, clinical observations, and chemical analysis providing support for the link between smoking and cancer (Kelley, 2020). Further, the Food and Drug Administration (FDA) took nearly half a century to make meaningful change from their 1963 declaration that tobacco products were harmless until the Family Smoking Prevention and Tobacco Control Act of 2009 finally granted the FDA regulatory authority to oversee tobacco products at the federal level (Kelley, 2020).

Raising the legal drinking age to 21 is another example of a big "P" policy. In 1984, the United States raised the legal drinking age from 18 to 21 (Mann, 2000). Policymakers reviewed the evidence that the brain does not fully develop until the age of 21–25. Without a fully developed brain, individuals lack cognitive abilities to regulate their emotions and urges. With this policy change and increased age requirement, traffic fatalities decreased considerably (Volkow et al., 2017).

A small "p" policy led by a grassroots organization and supported at the federal, state, local, and tribal level is the Mothers Against Drunk Driving (MADD) campaign. MADD has been effective in preventing and reducing alcohol misuse and related consequences. MADD utilized a public health approach to change attitudes about drinking and driving in the United States. A recent poll by the Gallup Organization reports that 94% of people know about MADD (Fell & Voas, 2006). MADD efforts resulted in a significant reduction in alcohol-related traffic deaths (from 30,000 in 190 to 16,694 in 2004) (Fell & Voas, 2006).

Bowen and Zwi's evidence-based decision-making framework based on the *diffusion of innovation* theory is a starting point for considering how policies are developed (Bowen & Zwi, 2005). Within the policy model (Figure 6.3), there are conditions at the individual, organizational, and systems level that impact policy uptake. In Chapter 2, we discussed evidence-based on IOM's standards, SAMHSA's standards, and the Cochrane Review. These would be considered **research evidence. Knowledge and ideas** is another form of evidence and results from workgroups, published reports, practice documents, the internet, and resources developed by a treatment program or evaluation. **Politics** create the third type of evidence where ideas and interests are generated from government agendas, political parties, opportunities, emergencies, and marketing. **Economics** is the fourth type of evidence that may be considered in policymaking. Economic evidence from a CEA of CBA evaluation might demonstrate a program is cost-effective (see Chapter 3) or has the potential to bring in revenue and opportunity to support continued programming and treatment. The strongest predictor of evidence use in policy is politics and economic

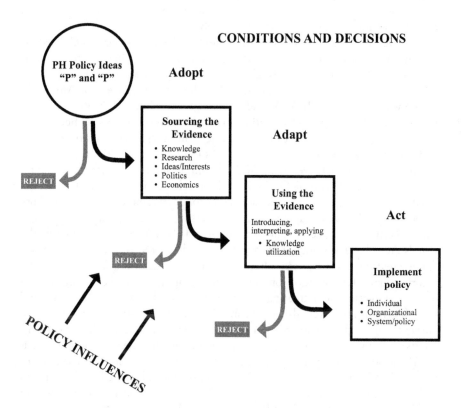

Figure 6.3 Policy Informed by Evidence.

considerations. Using evidence is based on how it is introduced, interpreted, and applied to a given problem (or in some cases a wicked public health problem). Take the example of smoking inside casinos. There is sufficient research evidence to suggest it is harmful to public health and exposure increases the risk of heart attacks, heart disease, lung cancer, and a variety of other cancers. Sufficient knowledge and information suggest that Smokefree Indoor Air (SFIA) laws are the most effective approach to protecting the public from secondhand smoke (Centers for Disease Control and Prevention, n.d.; Cheng et al., 2011). Yet politics and economics (the strongest predictors of evidence use) are likely the reason for stalled policy efforts. Until these two are addressed, there is no amount of evidence or knowledge that really matters time for change.

Federal Policies

There are multiple big "P" policies that may be considered when evaluating treatment programs using a public health approach perspective. Box 6.1 outlines some big "P" policies related to patient records, disclosures, and more.

The next section explains how these big "P" policies relate to treatment program settings (note this is not a comprehensive list).

The **Mental Health Parity and Addiction Equity Act of 2008** (MHPAEA) and the **Affordable Care Act of 2010** (ACA) now allow primary care providers to treat SUD like any other disease. However, a 2014 report published by the American Psychological Association (APA) found that just 4% of Americans were aware of the MHPAEA and their rights for mental health coverage (American Psychological Association, n.d.). More recently, researchers report increases in access to services and reductions in emergency department visits and hospital stays because of these two acts (Volkow et al., 2017).

The **21st Century Cures ACT of 2016** aims to improve health outcomes for individuals with MI and SUD who have been released from prison (Cole et al., 2018). Importantly the Cures Act advocates for decriminalizing substance abuse through a public health approach and addressing racial disparities that plague the US criminal justice system. While beyond the scope of this chapter, the Cure's Act objectives align with a public health approach, some examples include creating court-ordered alternatives to incarceration, creating mental health courses for low-level offenders, increasing access to behavioral health services, targeting, and treating individuals with a history of MI, SUD, and homelessness. This Act also established residential treatment programs and grants for individuals with co-occurring disorders. Funding for drug treatment courts and alternative incarceration programs, mental health training, crisis intervention, and training for criminal justice and law enforcement is also included. The Cure's Act is an example of a multi-pronged public health approach to SUD because it addresses current policies, systems, and environments that need to change for public health. Research on the impact of the Cure's Act is

---

Box 6.1   Federal Laws Related to Treatment Programs

SUPPORT Act
21st Century Cures Act
Comprehensive Addiction and Recovery Act (CARA)
Affordable Care Act (ACA)
Tribal Law and Order Act (TLOA)
Mental Health Parity and Addiction Equity Act
Americans with Disabilities Act (ADA)
Sober Truth on Preventing (STOP) Underage Drinking Act
Garret Lee Smith Memorial Act
Children's Health Act

---

mixed, where some feel that it has made a difference and others cite language issues, funding shortfalls, and unrealistic expectations (Barlas, 2018).

The **Substance Use-Disorder Prevention that Promotes Opioid Recovery and Treatment for Patients and Communities Act of 2018 (SUPPORT)** aims to address the nations opioid crisis. Key provisions in the Act include State Targeted Response Grants (STR), first responder training, comprehensive opioid recovery centers, best practices for recovery housing, and common indicators to identify fraudulent recovery housing operators (Substance Abuse and Mental Health Services Administration, n.d). The Substance Abuse Prevention and Treatment Block Grant (SABG) is an example of a big "P" policy mandated by law to provide funding and technical assistance for substance misuse services (Ballard et al., 2021). Grant funds awarded to all 50 states and beyond require that states use at least 20% of their funding for primary prevention. For more information on policies related to MHSU, check out the Resources section at the end of this chapter.

Accrediting Bodies and Treatment Program Policy Examples

Treatment programs must follow federal policies and practice guidelines that are driven by various accreditation bodies. While beyond the scope of this chapter or text, examples of these include the Commission on Accreditation of Rehabilitation Facilities (CARF) and the Joint Commission on Accreditation of Healthcare Organizations (JACHO). Treatment programs develop policies and procedures to meet accreditation requirements, these are considered small "p" policies. One Level II intensive outpatient treatment program has a policy and procedure guide that includes topics such as program services provided, governing body, program reporting, fiduciary and fiscal management, and human resource management.

Within this small "p" treatment program policy, big "P" policies are cited such as compliance with 42 CFR, Part 2 Federal Confidentiality, 45 CFR Part 160 and 164, Health Insurance Portability and Accountability Act (HIPAA), and other legal restrictions affecting the confidentiality of alcohol and drug abuse client records. In addition, policies include regulatory, licensure, and accreditation certification, ethical codes of conduct, cultural competency and diversity plan, community involvement and collaboration, information technology and social media, quality assurance, strategic planning, risk management, and annual reporting requirements.

State Policy Examples

Prescription Drug Monitoring Program Policy Example

The Centers for Disease Control Prescription Drug Monitoring Program (PDMP) is an example of a big "P" policy that was implemented at the state level throughout US. PDMPs are databases that collect data on opioid misuse, OUD, and overdose. Notably, PDMPs increased public health access to data that would allow faster response and prevention to opioid-related harms (Davis et al., 2021). Rhodes and colleagues conducted a systematic review of PDMPs and impacts from implementation, they found limited evidence that PDMPs reduced opioid-related consequences and harms. Authors point to the overall value of PDMPs and regulating opioid prescribing (Rhodes et al., 2019). For more information on PDMPs check out the Resources section at the end of this chapter.

Missouri Medication First Model

Missouri created a Medication First treatment approach for addressing OUD modeled after the Housing First model (described later in this Chapter). This model was supported by the 21st Century Cures Act, Pub. L. 144–255.51 The key principles of Medication First are:

1. People with OUD People with OUD receive pharmacotherapy treatment as quickly as possible, prior to lengthy assessments or treatment planning sessions.
2. Maintenance pharmacotherapy is delivered without arbitrary tapering or time limits.
3. Individualized psychosocial services are continually offered but not required as a condition of pharmacotherapy.
4. Pharmacotherapy is discontinued only if it is worsening the person's condition.

Missouri reports that 69 treatment sites are implementing Medication First principles (State of Missouri, 2021). More than 10,000 people have received treatment and outcomes demonstrate that the model promotes greater adherence to evidence-based medication for the treatment of OUD, more timely access to medication, improved retention, and cost savings associated with fewer reimbursable services.

California Department of Health Care Services ACES Aware Initiative

California is leading the way with a comprehensive ACES Aware Initiative that promotes trauma screenings and trauma-informed care for providers. Providers are encouraged to attend the training to understand more about a patient's health risk due to toxic stress while promoting a trauma-informed approach, a big "P" policy. Screenings are now covered by Medi-Cal for children and adults (California Department of Health Care Services, 2021). For screening tools and more information on ACES, check out the Resources section at the end of this chapter.

Oregon Health Authority Establishes Standards for Addiction

The Oregon Health Authority established standards for addiction services under the Health Systems Division Chapter 415. These small "p" policies were developed by OHA and include standards for licensing and procedures for various addiction-related topics including gambling, opioid abuse, alcohol detoxification, recovery, driving under the influence of intoxicants, restricted licenses, substance abuse prevention, standards for the Oregon Department of Corrections, and health professionals' services and licensing (Oregon Secretary of State, n.d.). Some policies are specific to treatment programs, for example, their **Standards for Outpatient Treatment Programs, OAR 415-020-0015**. OHA standards include administrative requirements that outline reimbursement for opioid treatment services, policies and procedures for outpatient opioid treatment program operations, personnel policies, rules for staff, standards of program staff use of alcohol or other drugs, compliance with federal and state personnel regulations, personnel records, confidentiality and retention, disabilities act compliance, insurance, and prevention.

Oregon Decriminalizes Drugs

I am an Oregonian. I live here and I love it. But, Oregon has experienced some of the greatest challenges when it comes to addressing MHSUD. Access to treatment for drug addiction in Oregon is the worst in the nation (all 50 states, for individuals 12 and older). In 2018, law enforcement officers in Oregon arrested 8,881 people having drugs in their possession (Oregon Health Authority, n.d.). Oregon arrested and convicted African Americans for cocaine possession at a rate that was 100 times higher than Whites in 2015. These egregious acts led Oregon to draft Measure 110, the Drug Addiction Treatment and Recovery Act.

This Act was passed in November 2020 and makes health assessments, treatment, and recovery services available for all people who want or need access to these services. Importantly this Act removes criminal penalties for low-level drug possession (Oregon Health Authority, n.d.) and if police find lesser amounts of illegal drugs on someone or in a vehicle they are subject to a $100 fine. The person can either pay the fine or waive the fine and attend a health screening. The Oregon Health Authority was tasked with funding treatment and recovery services through addiction recovery centers and community access to care grants. The Act required 15 addiction recovery centers open every day of the week and hour to open by October 1, 2021. Grants to support addiction recovery centers, community-based services, a 24/7 telephone addiction recovery center, and an oversight and accountability council were established as a result of this Act.

Although these big "P" and small "p" policies indicate movement towards broad understanding and support for effective evidence-based public health and a focus on quality of care, there is still work to be done. Researchers call for education about the factors that place individuals at risk for developing SUD (genetic, age-related, and environmental factors) and developing policies and interventions that address the SDOH (Aas et al., 2021; Cole et al., 2018; Volkow et al., 2017). A systems change approach provides a path forward for potentially improving research, policy, and outcomes.

Systems Change

Systems Change is the process of improving the capacity and service delivery of systems to improve access, and/or quality for people in a community. Examples include developing plans or implementing new interventions or processes within a treatment program setting, adapting existing models for a client population, utilizing new technologies such as telehealth, or creating training opportunities for staff and partners. The current health model is focused on a disease-treatment approach, where individuals with MHSUD (or other diseases) are treated with medicine and expected to recover. This is a parameter of the current system. The disease-treatment model approach is rewarded by big pharmaceutical companies, high insurance premiums for specialists, and results in wait times that are not realistic or feasible. The current system fails to fully support recovery-based systems of care, but there are some examples of systems change that give me hope. Trauma-informed approaches to treatment and recovery are one of the most widely accepted and implemented systems change approaches within a treatment setting.

Trauma-Informed Systems Change

SAMHSA advocates for trauma-informed systems and defines trauma-informed systems change as, "A program, organization or system is trauma-informed when it realizes the widespread impact of trauma and understands potential paths for recovery; recognizes the signs and symptoms of trauma in clients, families, staff, and others involved with the system; responds by fully integrating knowledge about trauma into policies, procedures, and practices; and seeks to actively resist retraumatization." SAMHSA identified system principles of a trauma-informed approach (Substance Abuse and Mental Health Services Administration, 2018, p. 1.).

1. Safety
2. Trustworthiness and transparency
3. Peer support
4. Collaboration and mutuality
5. Empowerment, voice, and choice
6. Cultural, historical, and gender issues (2018)

Culturally Centered and Culturally Sensitive Systems Change

Within various federal funding programs, grants are required to address the National Culturally and Linguistically Appropriate Services (CLAS) in Health and Health Care (US Department of Health and Human Services, n.d.). Standards were designed to advance health equity, improve quality, and eliminate health disparities covering four domains: 1) principal standards, 2) governance, leadership, and workforce, 3) communication and language assistance, and 4) engagement, continuous improvement, and accountability. While federal grants are required to attend to CLAS standards, their operationalization of these standards is not well understood. Take the **CLAS standards** example from a recent treatment program proposal to SAMSHA.

All proposed activities of the project will adhere to the National Standards for CLAS. Because the focus of the project is working with a tribal community with unique traditions and languages, it is critical to comply with these standards. All proposed staff and partners have experience both personally and professionally with tribal communities and can provide effective, equitable, understandable, and respectful quality care, as outlined in the Principal Standard of CLAS. The project will ensure culturally appropriate implementation of the project's activities and will provide culturally appropriate media materials that are not only tribally specific but easy to understand in both written language and imagery (Kelley, 2019). This summary outlines how a program will attend to CLAS standards but does not provide an accountability framework to ensure that CLAS standards are upheld.

Dutta's work on health communication in cultural settings furthers understanding about the application of culture within a given context. Another term to describe cultural adaptations and approaches within a health care setting is a culturally sensitive approach. Dutta distinguishes culturally sensitive approaches and culturally centered approaches, where a culturally sensitive approach is based on values, beliefs, and practices within a community (2007). In contrast, a culturally centered approach views culture as a complex and dynamic system with constructed and varied meanings based on a given culture, history, and local, state, federal influences (Dutta, 2007). Both cultural sensitivity and culturally centered approaches require systems change to address power structures, ideals, and values that may be different within cultures, staff, clients, and treatment settings.

Public Health Takeaway—Creating or requiring standards that address culture, language, and context are a starting point. But standards fail to hold systems accountable.

Recovery-Oriented Systems of Care and Systems Change

You might recall that in Chapter 4 we reviewed ROSCs and we will briefly describe how these relate to systems change. ROSCs create a system of care for individuals with MHSUD and their families. One example of a systems change that came from the ROSC movement is the recovery support services (RSS). RSS provides a continuum of care, including greater access to treatment, childcare and transportation, education, employment, and housing. Some ROSC systems are attempting to address social determinants of behavioral health conditions. Others are focused on developing a citizenship-oriented approach that promotes community connections and self-actualization (Davidson et al., 2021).

Peer Recovery Support as Systems Change

Peer recovery support and peer coaching approaches are other examples of how the current treatment shifted from a purely clinically focused system to a community and peer recovery system. Extant evaluation and research have documented the impacts and effectiveness of peer recovery support (Kelley et al., 2021). The Association for Addiction Professionals established requirements for peer recovery support specialist certification, eligibility, application, and renewal (https://www.naadac.org/ncprss). A major milestone in the implementation of PRS models is the certification of peer support specialists which standardized the certification process for peer support specialists and allowed for third-party billing of PRS services. Eddie and colleagues conducted a systematic review of peer recovery support services and coaching, they found that this approach reduces substance use and SUD relapse rates, increases social supports and supportive relationships with treatment providers, and helps individuals with SUD advantage systems of recovery (Eddie et al., 2019).

Environmental Change

A healing forest is what David Moore and Don Coyhis describe when writing about the environment and conditions that people need to heal. The healing forest model recognizes that change occurs at the individual level, but this change is driven by environmental factors. They espouse that change is best supported within an environment that is seeded with the resources to foster personal growth and active involvement in a community (Moore & Coyhis, 2010). Environmental systems change may also include economic and social conditions that impact treatment and recovery outcomes.

Housing First

Housing First models are a recovery-oriented systems change approach to address homelessness that are based on the concept that all people deserve housing and that in order to recover, people need adequate housing. Principles guiding the Housing First models are as follows:

1. Immediate access to permanent housing with no housing readiness requirements
2. Consumer choice and self-determination
3. Recovery orientation
4. Individualized and client-driven supports
5. Social and community Integration (Smith, 2021)

Tsai reviewed the evidence in support of the Housing First model and reported that it resulted in greater improvements in housing outcomes for homeless adults (2020). In this review, he identified four RCTs of the Housing First model and one RCT conducted with five cities in Canada. Results from the Canadian RCT show that Housing First participants were in stable housing 73% of the time compared with control participants, who were in stable housing just 32% of the time (Tsai, 2020).

Recovery Housing

Recovery housing and sober living houses are part of a healing forest concept, however, not all forests are created equally with the same risk and protective factors in place. Mericle and colleagues reviewed sober living houses in Los Angeles and utilized neighborhood sociodemographic, alcohol outlets, treatment and recovery resources, accessibility (walking score). Sober living houses were close to treatment and recovery resources (this was considered protective), but the majority were not located in a walkable area (this may impact access to employment and education) (Mericle et al., 2019).

Diehl Reis and Laranjeira describe a halfway house in Jardim Angela in the city of São Paulo/SP, Brazil (2008). This house was located in a neighborhood with one of the highest violence rates in the world. With 10-beds, this facility was open for individuals with AUD for up to 30 days and served 130 people from 1999 to 2001. Created with a comfortable and community atmosphere, this halfway house upheld health, social support networks, and abstinence. A communitarian agent stayed at the house 24 hours a day and assisted with various tasks such as meal preparation, games, personal hygiene, recovery activities, and family communications. Psychiatric, psychological, nursing, and social assistance services were provided twice per week at an outpatient center near the halfway house. Volunteers from Jardim Angela taught yoga, arts, and horticulture. The cost was minimal (although this is 20 years ago), but just $13.00 per day including meals, medications, and supports. Researchers and advocates of this community-based, environmental change approach call attention to the cost-effectiveness, and the long-term positive impacts of building social support and networks for individuals in recovery (Reis & Laranjeira, 2008).

Drug Consumption Rooms/Supervised Injection Facilities

A harm reduction approach is an example of environmental change. Canada is leading the world in supervised injection facilities (SIF) and opened the first SIF in 2003 (Kerr et al., 2017). Extant evidence demonstrates that SIFs reduce health and social harms associated with injection drug use. Health Canada opened the first SIF in 2003 with federal approval granted by the Health Minister. SIF's first site included 13 spaces for injection and open up to 24 hours per day. Insite developers agreed to rigorously evaluate the pilot program to determine whether it reduced public disorder, infectious disease transmission, and overdose. A secondary goal of Insite was to refer individuals to external programs such as detoxification and treatment. The pilot evaluation demonstrated that the harm reduction approach was effective in reaching these goals. Findings from the pilot evaluation found no increases in crime or initiation of injection drugs linked to the SIF intervention (Kerr et al., 2017). There are two critical issues with harm reduction evaluation and implementation moving forward. First, evaluation methods that assess harm reduction approaches are varied, with some using an ecological study design, others modeling techniques, cohorts, cross-sectional surveys, or service records (Belackova et al., 2019). Consistent evaluation methods and standards may contribute to a more robust evidence-based and address stigma and misperceptions around harm reduction models. Second, political opposition to harm reduction models has been noted in Canada and other locations implementing a harm reduction approach. Advocates of harm reduction approaches call for greater awareness and outreach, policy change, and peer-implemented harm reduction models (Belackova et al., 2019; Kerr et al., 2017).

Policy, systems, and environmental (PSE) change provide an opportunity to target change at the individual, family, community, organizational, or systems level. When considering what to change it is essential to engage partners, members of the target population (clients, staff, families, others), in the planning process. Consider the theory of change (ToC) from Chapter 3, the kinds of inputs, outputs, and outcomes that you envision happening from your work. Prioritize the needs of populations who have historically been underrepresented, marginalized, stigmatized, or othered. Consider needs assessments, environmental scans, document reviews, literature reviews, or other forms of information gathering to inform the process (see Chapter 5). Readiness for change is huge. Recall the example earlier in this Chapter describing smoking policies inside gaming facilities. Despite undeniable evidence that secondhand smoke is deleterious to public health, the readiness for change at the political and economic levels is missing. Readiness for change at the individual level is also required (see Chapter 2). Once PSEs are implemented, do not forget to evaluate their impacts, consider the critical evaluation question, "How did it work?"

Addressing barriers to policy implementation might be the next big step for mankind and public health. Brownson and colleagues identified barriers to evidence-based public health policy. I know we cannot focus only on the barriers, but moving public health forward requires we define what the problems are (step 1). With these barriers outlined in Figure 6.4, here are some potential solutions. Process solutions could include fast data preparation and dissemination and finding new ways to communicate data. Content solutions could include identifying essential components of policy interventions and what is needed to move forward while using multiple tools, borrowed from researchers and evaluators, to determine cost-effectiveness, impact, and access. Outcome solutions could focus on developing systems policy for surveillance (step 1) and

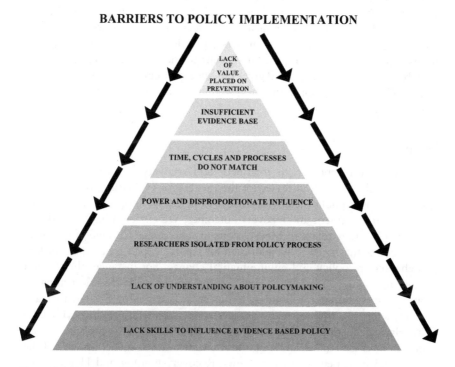

BARRIERS TO POLICY IMPLEMENTATION

LACK OF VALUE PLACED ON PREVENTION

INSUFFICIENT EVIDENCE BASE

TIME, CYCLES AND PROCESSES DO NOT MATCH

POWER AND DISPROPORTIONATE INFLUENCE

RESEARCHERS ISOLATED FROM POLICY PROCESS

LACK OF UNDERSTANDING ABOUT POLICYMAKING

LACK SKILLS TO INFLUENCE EVIDENCE BASED POLICY

Figure 6.4 Barriers to Policy Implementation.

(Source: Adapted from Brownson, 2009).

utilizing multiple forms of evidence to determine what works, for whom, and why (Brownson et al., 2009).

Where Are We and Where Do We Need to Go?

We have come a long way, but we have more to do. The United States spends more than $10,000 per person each year on healthcare, this is double than other developed nations—funding in the United States has been diverted to private healthcare companies and systems, leaving out the most vulnerable (Los Angeles Times, 2020). Health inequities persist. The greatest disappointment is that we have not addressed the systemic and structural issues that divide individuals, families, communities, and nations, even though we have the evidence (Bowen & Zwi, 2005). Not all children born today are given the same opportunities as their peers. Underlying factors contributing to health inequities, such as poverty, inadequate housing, education, and systemic racism have not been fully addressed. Until we address the underlying causes of health inequities, nothing will change that much. Policy change (uptake, adoption, and implementation) is one of the most effective ways to address wicked problems. **The Health in All Policies (HiAP)** approach may be a potential solution. Developed in the late 1990s by the Finnish government, HiAP aims to develop public policies that systematically address health outcomes and health systems. HiAP considers the implications of decisions made, seeks opportunities for synergy, and avoids negative impacts on health. Grounded in principles of health equity and human rights, HiAP aims to increase accountability in policymaking (Leppo, 2013). HiAP gives me hope that change is possible, that we can shift the needle, transform the paradigm, turn on the light ... but it is getting dark out here.

Wrap-up

A public health approach to treatment and recovery can be effective. We started this chapter with a review of the process for evaluating treatment programs utilizing a public health approach. Policies, systems, and environments contribute to treatment and recovery outcomes. We explored big "P" and little "p" policies as they relate to MHSU domains and discussed some of the major gaps in policy that need to be addressed for equity. Topics that stand out from this chapter are policy and environmental change. For instance, the decriminalization of drugs—we learned that Oregon passed a law that decriminalizes small amounts of drugs. Preliminary results show that passing this law increased recovery supports, systems, and outcomes for persons who use drugs (PWUD). Win! Harm reduction models also support a public health approach and outcomes from these studies show significant benefits with reductions in risk behaviors and increased access for clients. Recovery housing and Housing First models demonstrate the power of environment and social conditions on recovery outcomes. As a basic human right, advocates of Housing First and recovery homes call for improved policy, access, self-determination, and social integration as the path forward.

The last thought is about trauma. Trauma must be addressed if we are going to make any headway in the field of public health, addiction, treatment, and recovery. Unresolved trauma is pervasive with MHSUD populations (>80%) and attempts to prevent ACEs through comprehensive screenings and training are a step in the right direction. California is leading the way with its ACEs Aware Initiative that promotes screening and trains providers in trauma-informed care principles and practices. Go California!

Discussion Questions

1. When you think about a public health approach to treatment and recovery, what is most important?
2. Consider the Policy, Systems, and Environment (PSE) model and the examples presented in this chapter, which are likely to have the greatest public health benefits?
3. Describe the reasons why people might criticize harm reduction approaches and drug consumption? What are some potential ways that public health advocates can address these criticisms and stigmatization?
4. If you had to select one theory that explains addiction, treatment, and how people recover, what would you select? The Rat Park experiment and theory of human behavior? The disease model of addiction? The choice model? What about other theories and approaches covered in Chapter 2?

Resources

Public Health Approach Resources

American Public Health Association, Health In All Policies, https://www.apha.org/topics-and-issues/health-in-all-policies

California ACES Aware, https://www.dhcs.ca.gov/provgovpart/Pages/TraumaCare.aspx

Centers for Disease Control OD2A, https://www.cdc.gov/drugoverdose/od2a/index.html

Centers for Disease Control, HIAP https://www.cdc.gov/policy/hiap/index.htm

Centers for Disease Control Drug Overdose Prescription Drug Monitoring Programs https://www.cdc.gov/drugoverdose/pdmp/index.html

Code of Federal Regulations, https://www.ecfr.gov/

Harm Reduction Principles for Healthcare Settings, https://link.springer.com/article/10.1186/s12954-017-0196-4

Institute for Health Metrics and Evaluation (IHME) Measuring What Matters: http://www.healthdata.org/gbd/faq

Substance Abuse and Mental Health Services Administration Trauma Informed in Care in Behavioral Health Services, https://store.samhsa.gov/sites/default/files/d7/priv/sma15–4420.pdf

Pew Charitable Trust Imprisonment and Drugs, https://www.pewtrusts.org/en/research-and-analysis/issue-briefs/2018/03/more-imprisonment-does-not-reduce-state-drug-problems

Prevention Institute, Tools for Primary Prevention and Health Equity, https://www.preventioninstitute.org/focus-areas

Substance Abuse and Mental Health Services Administration Laws and Regulations related to substance abuse and mental health: https://www.samhsa.gov/about-us/who-we-are/laws-regulations

The Community Guide, https://www.thecommunityguide.org/

Trauma Resource Institute, Building Resilience Awakening Hope, https://www.traumaresourceinstitute.com/home

Understanding the Mental Health Parity Act: https://www.nami.org/Your-Journey/Individuals-with-Mental-Illness/Understanding-Health-Insurance/What-is-Mental-Health-Parity

World Health Organization, Health in All Policies Introduction, https://www.euro.who.int/__data/assets/pdf_file/0007/188809/Health-in-All-Policies-final.pdf

References

Aas, C. F., Vold, J. H., Gjestad, R., Skurtveit, S., Lim, A. G., Gjerde, K. V., Løberg, E.-M., Johansson, K. A., & Fadnes, L. T., for the INTRO-HCV Study Group. (2021). Substance use and symptoms of mental health disorders: A prospective cohort of patients with severe substance use disorders in Norway. *Substance Abuse Treatment, Prevention and Policy*, 16, 1–10. 10.1186/s13011-021-00354-1

Alegría, M., Frank, R. G., Hansen, H. B., Sharfstein, J. M., Shim, R. S., & Tierney, M. (2021). Transforming mental health and addiction services. *Health Affairs*, 40(2), 226–234. 10.1377/hlthaff.2020.01472

Alexander, B. K., Coambs, R. B., & Hadaway, P. F. (1978). The effect of housing and gender on morphine self-administration in rats. *Psychopharmacology*, 58(2), 175–179. 10.1007/BF00426903

American Psychological Association (n.d.) *Few Americans aware of their rights for mental health coverage*. https://Www.Apa.Org. Retrieved November 2, 2021, from https://www.apa.org/news/press/releases/2014/05/mental-health-coverage

Americans with Disabilities Act (n.d.). *Questions and Answers*. Retrieved November 2, 2021, from https://www.ada.gov/employmt.htm

Ballard, P. J., Pankratz, M., Wagoner, K. G., Cornacchione Ross, J., Rhodes, S. D., Azagba, S., Song, E. Y., & Wolfson, M. (2021). Changing course: Supporting a shift to environmental strategies in a state prevention system. *Substance Abuse Treatment, Prevention, and Policy*, 16(1), 7. 10.1186/s13011-020-00341-y

Bao, Y., Williams, A. R., & Schackman, B. R. (2020). COVID-19 can change the way we respond to the opioid crisis – For the better. *Psychiatric Services (Washington, D.C.)*, 71(12), 1214–1215. 10.1176/appi.ps.202000226

Barlas, S. (2018). The 21st century cures act: FDA implementation one year later. *Pharmacy and Therapeutics*, 43(3), 149–179. https://www.ncbi.nlm.nih.gov/pmc/articles/PMC5821241/

Belackova, V., Salmon, A. M., Day, C. A., Ritter, A., Shanahan, M., Hedrich, D., Kerr, T., & Jauncey, M. (2019). Drug consumption rooms: A systematic review of evaluation methodologies. *Drug and Alcohol Review*, 38(4), 406–422. 10.1111/dar.12919

Bethell, C. D., Solloway, M. R., Guinosso, S., Hassink, S., Srivastav, A., Ford, D., & Simpson, L. A. (2017). Prioritizing possibilities for child and family health: An agenda to address adverse childhood experiences and foster the social and emotional roots of well-being in pediatrics. *Academic Pediatrics*, 17(7), S36–S50. 10.1016/j.acap.2017.06.002

Borden, T. (2016). *Every 25 seconds—The human toll of criminalizing drug use in the United States*. Human Rights Watch.

Bowen, S., & Zwi, A. B. (2005). Pathways to "evidence-informed" policy and practice: A framework for action. *PLoS Medicine*, 2(7), e166. 10.1371/journal.pmed.0020166

Brownley, J. (2021). *Text - H.R.1329 - 117th Congress (2021–2022): Surface Transportation Investment Act of 2021 (2021/2022) [Legislation]*. https://www.congress.gov/bill/117th-congress/house-bill/1329/text

Brownson, R. C., Chriqui, J. F., & Stamatakis, K. A. (2009). Understanding evidence-based public health policy. *American Journal of Public Health*, 99(9), 1576–1583. 10.2105/AJPH.2008.156224

CADCA (2018). *Addressing the opioid crisis through community prevention: An Application of the Seven Strategies for Community Change. Practical Theorist*. https://njprevent.com/wp-content/uploads/2018/09/cadcapracticaltheorist.pdf

California Department of Health Care Services (2021). *Trauma Screenings and Trauma-Informed Care Provider Trainings*. California.gov. https://www.dhcs.ca.gov/provgovpart/Pages/TraumaCare.aspx

Centers for Disease Control and Prevention. (n.d.). *State Tobacco Activities Tracking and Evaluation (STATE) System*. Centers for Disease Control and Prevention. Retrieved November 13, 2021, from https://www.cdc.gov/statesystem/factsheets/gaming/Gaming.html

Chandler, R. K., Fletcher, B. W., & Volkow, N. D. (2009). Treating drug abuse and addiction in the criminal justice system: Improving public health and safety. *JAMA: The Journal of the American Medical Association*, 301(2), 183–190. 10.1001/jama.2008.976

Cheng, K.-W., Glantz, S. A., & Lightwood, J. M. (2011). Association between smokefree laws and voluntary smokefree-home rules. *American Journal of Preventive Medicine*, 41(6), 566–572. 10.1016/j.amepre.2011.08.014

Cole, D. M., Thomas, D. M., Field, K., Wool, A., Lipiner, T., Massenberg, N., & Guthrie, B. J. (2018). The 21st century cures act implications for the reduction of racial health disparities in the US criminal justice system: A public health approach. *Journal of Racial and Ethnic Health Disparities*, 5(4), 885–893. 10.1007/s40615-017-0435-0

Davidson, L., Rowe, M., DiLeo, P., Bellamy, C., & Delphin-Rittmon, M. (2021). Recovery-oriented systems of care: A perspective on the past, present, and future. *Alcohol Research: Current Reviews*, 41(1), 09. 10.35946/arcr.v41.1.09

Davis, C., Sargent, S., Vick, J., Kuoh, H., & Cote, P. (2021). *Leveraging Prescription Drug Monitoring Program (PDMP) Data in Overdose Prevention and Response*. 33. https://www.cdc.gov/drugoverdose/pdf/Leveraging-PDMPs-508.pdf

Des Jarlais, D. C. (2017). Harm reduction in the USA: The research perspective and an archive to David Purchase. *Harm Reduction Journal*, 14(1), 51. 10.1186/s12954-017-0178-6

Dutta, M. J. (2007). Communicating about culture and health: Theorizing culture-centered and cultural sensitivity approaches. *Communication Theory*, *17*(3), 304–328. 10.1111/j.1468-2885.2007.00297.x

Eddie, D., Hoffman, L., Vilsaint, C., Abry, A., Bergman, B., Hoeppner, B., Weinstein, C., & Kelly, J. F. (2019). Lived experience in new models of care for substance use disorder: A systematic review of peer recovery support services and recovery coaching. *Frontiers in Psychology*, *10*, 1052. 10.3389/fpsyg.2019.01052

Fell, J. C., & Voas, R. B. (2006). Mothers against drunk driving (MADD): The first 25 years. *Traffic Injury Prevention*, *7*(3), 195–212. 10.1080/15389580600727705

Gage, S. H., & Sumnall, H. R. (2019). Rat park: How a rat paradise changed the narrative of addiction. *Addiction*, *114*(5), 917–922. 10.1111/add.14481

Garcia, J. (2020). H.R. 6637 - 116th Congress (2019–2020): Health Equity and Accountability Act of 2020 [Legislation]. https://www.congress.gov/bill/116th-congress/house-bill/6637/text

Gibbs, B. R., Lytle, R., & Wakefield, W. (2019). Outcome effects on recidivism among drug court participants. *Criminal Justice and Behavior*, *46*(1), 115–135. 10.1177/0093 854818800528

Grabbe, L., & Miller-Karas, E. (2017). The trauma resiliency model: A "bottom-up" intervention for trauma psychotherapy. *Journal of the American Psychiatric Nurses Association*, *24*, 107839031774513. 10.1177/1078390317745133

Harm Reduction Principles (n.d.). *National Harm Reduction Coalition*. Retrieved November 12, 2021, from https://harmreduction.org/about-us/principles-of-harm-reduction/

Henry, B. F., Mandavia, A. D., Paschen-Wolff, M. M., Hunt, T., Humensky, J. L., Wu, E., Pincus, H. A., Nunes, E. V., Levin, F. R., & El-Bassel, N. (2020). COVID-19, mental health, and opioid use disorder: Old and new public health crises intertwine. *Psychological Trauma: Theory, Research, Practice and Policy*, *12*(Suppl 1), S111–S112. 10.1037/tra0000660

H.R.6637 - 116th Congress *(2019–2020): Health Equity and Accountability Act of 2020* (2019/2020). (2020, July 9) [Webpage]. https://www.congress.gov/bill/116th-congress/house-bill/6637/text

Institute of Medicine (2012). *For the Public's Health: Investing in a Healthier Future*. National Academies Press (US). 10.17226/13268

International Society for Traumatic Stress Studies (2015). *A Public Health Approach to Trauma: Implications for Science, Practice, Policy, and the Role of ISTSS*. https://istss.org/getattachment/Education-Research/White-Papers/A-Public-Health-Approach-to-Trauma/Trauma-and-PH-Task-Force-Report.pdf.aspx

Kelley, A. (2019). Unpublished report, CLAS Standards for SAMHSA Grant Application.

Kelley, A. (2020). *Public Health Evaluation and the Social Determinants of Health* (Vol. 1–1 online resource [xi, 178 pages]: illustrations, maps). Routledge, Taylor & Francis Group. https://www.taylorfrancis.com/books/9781003047810

Kelley, A., BigFoot, D., Small, C., Mexicancheyenne, T., & Gondara, R. (2015). Recommendations from an American Indian reservation community-based suicide prevention program. *International Journal of Human Rights in Healthcare*, *8*(1), 3–13. 10.1108/IJHRH-10-2013-0025

Kelley, A., Restad, D., & Killsback, J. (2018). A public health approach: Documenting the risk and protective factors of suicide ideation in one American Indian community. *Psychological Services*, *15*(3), 325–331. 10.1037/ser0000211

Kelley, A., Steinberg, R., McCoy, T. P., Pack, R., & Pepion, L. (2021). Exploring recovery: Findings from a six-year evaluation of an American Indian peer recovery support program. *Drug and Alcohol Dependence, 221,* 108559. 10.1016/j.drugalcdep.2021.108559

Kerr, T., Mitra, S., Kennedy, M. C., & McNeil, R. (2017). Supervised injection facilities in Canada: Past, present, and future. *Harm Reduction Journal, 14*(1), 28. 10.1186/s12954-017-0154-1

Leppo, K. (Ed.). (2013). *Health in all policies: Seizing opportunities, implementing policies.* Ministry of Social Affairs and Health, Finland.

Lewis, M. (2017). Addiction and the brain: Development, not disease. *Neuroethics, 10,* 7–18 10.1007/s12152-016-9293-4

Los Angeles Times (2020). *It's not just coronavirus: America repeatedly fails at public health.* (2020, July 2). https://www.latimes.com/politics/story/2020-07-02/not-just-coronavirus-america-fails-public-health

Mann, K. (2000).One hundred years of alcoholism: The twentieth century. *Alcohol and Alcoholism, 35*(1), 10–15. 10.1093/alcalc/35.1.10

Marlatt, G. A. (1996). Harm reduction: Come as you are. *Addictive Behaviors, 21*(6), 779–788. 10.1016/0306-4603(96)00042-1

Mericle, A. A., Mahoney, E., Korcha, R., Delucchi, K., & Polcin, D. L. (2019). Sober living house characteristics: A multilevel analyses of factors associated with improved outcomes. *Journal of Substance Abuse Treatment, 98,* 28–38. 10.1016/j.jsat.2018.12.004

Moore, D., & Coyhis, D. (2010). The multicultural wellbriety peer recovery support program: Two decades of community-based recovery. *Alcoholism Treatment Quarterly, 28*(3), 273–292. 10.1080/07347324.2010.488530

National Academies of Science, Engineering, and Medicine (2020). *Promoting Positive Adolescent Health Behaviors and Outcomes: Thriving in the 21st Century.* Washington, DC: The National Academies Press. https://doi.org/10.17226/25552

National Institute on Drug Abuse (2020). *Criminal Justice DrugFacts. National Institute on Drug Abuse.* https://www.drugabuse.gov/publications/drugfacts/criminal-justice

Oregon Health Authority (n.d.). *Drug Addiction Treatment and Recovery Act: Behavioral Health Services: State of Oregon.* Retrieved November 12, 2021, from https://www.oregon.gov/oha/HSD/AMH/Pages/Measure110.aspx

Oregon Secretary of State (n.d.). *Administrative Rules.* Retrieved November 3, 2021, from https://secure.sos.state.or.us/oard/viewSingleRule.action?ruleVrsnRsn=103853

Pew Charitable Trust (2018). *More Imprisonment Does Not Reduce State Drug Problems.* Retrieved November 12, 2021, from http://pew.org/2tszeZl

Pickard, H. (2017). Responsibility without blame for addiction. *Neuroethics, 10*(1), 169–180. 10.1007/s12152-016-9295-2

Raffle, H., & Leach, V. (2020). *Adopting Collective Impact to Address the Opioid Epidemic.* Mental Health Ohio Addiction Services. http://npnconference.org/wp-content/uploads/2019/09/RAFFLE-LEACH-Adopting-Collective-Impact-NPN-8-27-245-400.pdf

Regis, C., Gaeta, J. M., Mackin, S., Baggett, T. P., Quinlan, J., & Taveras, E. M. (2020). Community care in reach: Mobilizing harm reduction and addiction treatment services for vulnerable populations. *Frontiers in Public Health, 8,* 501. 10.3389/fpubh.2020.00501

Reis, A. D., & Laranjeira, R. (2008). Halfway houses for alcohol dependents: From theoretical bases to implications for the organization of facilities. *Clinics (Sao Paulo, Brazil), 63*(6), 827–832. 10.1590/S1807-59322008000600020

Rhodes, E., Wilson, M., Robinson, A., Hayden, J. A., & Asbridge, M. (2019). The effectiveness of prescription drug monitoring programs at reducing opioid-related harms and consequences: A systematic review. *BMC Health Services Research, 19*(1), 784. 10.1186/s12913-019-4642-8

Smith, J. (2021). *Housing first model: An evidence-based approach to ending homelessness.* Heading Home Inc. https://www.headinghomeinc.org/housing-first-model/

State of Missouri (2021). *Medication First Approach.* https://www.nomodeaths.org/medication-first-implementation

Substance Abuse and Mental Health Services Administration (n.d.) *Laws and Regulations.* Retrieved November 2, 2021, from https://www.samhsa.gov/about-us/who-we-are/laws-regulations

Substance Abuse and Mental Health Services Administration (2011). *Current Statistics on the Prevalence and Characteristics of People Experiencing Homelessness in the United States.* https://www.samhsa.gov/sites/default/files/programs_campaigns/homelessness_programs_resources/hrc-factsheet-current-statistics-prevalence-characteristics-homelessness.pdf

Substance Abuse and Mental Health Services Administration, & Office of the Surgeon General. (2017). Vision for the future: A public health approach. In *Facing Addiction in America: The Surgeon General's Report on Alcohol, Drugs, and Health [Internet].* US Department of Health and Human Services. https://www.ncbi.nlm.nih.gov/books/NBK424861/

Substance Abuse and Mental Health Services Administration (2018). *SAMHSA's Trauma-Informed Approach: Key Assumptions and Principles Draft Document.* U.S. Department of Health and Human Services. https://www.nasmhpd.org/sites/default/files/TRAUMA-key_assumptions_and_principles_9-10-18.pdf

Tonko, P. (2019a). *H.R.2482 - 116th Congress (2019–2020): Mainstreaming Addiction Treatment Act of 2019 (2019/2020) [Legislation].* https://www.congress.gov/bill/116th-congress/house-bill/2482

Tonko, P. (2019b). *H.R.3925 - 116th Congress (2019–2020): Reducing Barriers to Substance Use Treatment Act (2019/2020) [Legislation].* https://www.congress.gov/bill/116th-congress/house-bill/3925

Tsai, J. (2020). Is the housing first model effective? Different evidence for different outcomes. *American Journal of Public Health, 110*(9), 1376. 10.2105/AJPH.2020.305835

US Department of Health and Human Services (n.d.). *National CLAS Standards.* https://thinkculturalhealth.hhs.gov/assets/pdfs/EnhancedNationalCLASStandards.pdf

U.S. Department of Housing and Urban Development (HUD) (n.d.). *Fair Housing: Rights and Obligations | HUD.gov /* Retrieved November 2, 2021, from https://www.hud.gov/program_offices/fair_housing_equal_opp/fair_housing_rights_and_obligations

Volkow, N. D. (2020). Collision of the COVID-19 and addiction epidemics. *Annals of Internal Medicine, 173*(1), 61–62. 10.7326/M20-1212

Volkow, N. D. (2021). Addiction should be treated, not penalized. *Neuropsychopharmacology, 46*(12), 2048–2050. 10.1038/s41386-021-01087-2

Volkow, N. D., Poznyak, V., Saxena, S., & Gerra, G. (2017). Drug use disorders: Impact of a public health rather than a criminal justice approach. *World Psychiatry, 16*(2), 213–214. 10.1002/wps.20428

7 The Message

CONTENTS

Learning Objectives

After reading this chapter, you should be able to

1. Discuss how to disseminate a recovery message using various platforms.
2. Describe the components of a communication strategy.
3. Summarize five key messages for a healing generation and the future of treatment program evaluation.
4. Discuss concepts of natural recovery and hope.

DOI: 10.4324/9781003290728-7

5. Discuss the gatekeeper myth, the role of treatment programs, and the implications of these in treatment and public health settings.

Communicating a Recovery Message

I have been wanting to write this book for a few years. The timing was not right. There is an unseen force in the writing process. One of my favorite authors Clarissa Pinkola Estes writes about a goblin in the wind, the unseen force behind a person's activities and creative life (2008, p. 519). I have felt the invisible unnamed powers throughout the writing process, and I am left with a few key messages that I must share before we close and celebrate the concluding chapter and its contents. If you read nothing else, read this chapter.

Up until now, we have focused on how to do an evaluation, what theories and research support treatment program efforts, and what evaluation looks like from a public health perspective (Chapter 6). We even created a framework for public health-focused evaluations in treatment settings, beginning with defining the problem, understanding the causes, evaluating the efforts, and promoting widespread adoption of what works (steps 1–4). There are challenges with promoting widespread adoption because even when evaluations create evidence that an intervention, policy, or approach is effective, evidence is not enough. Recall from Chapter 6 that we must also address politics and economic factors because these are the two primary drivers of evidence-based policy change.

Evaluations generate ideas, stories, evidence, understanding about what is happening in our world, what has value and meaning, what sticks and what does not, and what matters. Research does this too but in a different way. One of the key challenges that we have as evaluators is communicating the message. I mentioned in earlier chapters that we cannot just communicate everything to everyone, IRBs, directors, funding agencies—they all have a say in what goes out, and what stays in. So, we must check with them first, engage them in the communication process, and create a strategic communication and dissemination approach.

In my work, we have created various strategic plans, marketing plans, communication plans, risk communication plans, graphical abstracts, publications, reports, and more. We invest in a design team committed to health equity and create visual products that emphasize the primary message that people read. Previous texts have outlined examples of evaluation reports, strategies, infographics, and communications (Kelley, 2018, 2020). Here are some new examples that might help you as you think about communication and dissemination. I can tell you how to do it, but I would rather show you.

Not everyone wants to read a 100-page evaluation report. This past year we started using a graphical abstract template to communicate key results from evaluation efforts. Many journals require **graphical abstracts** to communicate the main findings of a research or evaluation article. A graphical abstract is one image (i.e., .jpg or .png) that combines all of the findings into one single designed document. Abstracts generally contain a title, background information, methods, findings, a conclusion, and reference or contact information. We developed a graphical abstract for the BRAVE study (Rushing et al., 2021) and an example of this graphical abstract is available here: https://mental.jmir.org/ 2021/9/e26158/. I utilize this same approach for evaluation findings from various treatment programs. Due to privacy issues, I cannot include these treatment program examples. In sum, graphical abstracts are an excellent way to promote a treatment program message or brand using print and online platforms.

Presenting data effectively is an entire discipline. There are rules to follow when considering how to communicate the findings of an evaluation utilizing both quantitative and qualitative data. One of my favorite resources for data visualization is Stephanie Evergreen. She provides online courses, workshops, and custom designs for evaluators and researchers. Check out the Resources section at the end of this chapter for more on data visualization.

We recently completed a project with a client that has a massive social media presence and following. They develop mHealth interventions (online) that reach American Indian youth and young adults throughout the United States and beyond. Here is a dissemination plan for an mHealth intervention. I've adapted some of the text in the plan for privacy.

The goal of this plan was to facilitate the mHealth intervention in communities throughout the United States. The client and dissemination partners are the **source**. The **message** is that the mHealth intervention works, it can be used in a variety of settings, and just about anyone can lead the intervention with the help of the Facilitators Guide. The **audience** includes healthcare professionals, schools, and individuals working with young people aged 15–24; specifically, health departments, church groups, schools, colleges and universities, youth leadership programs, youth treatment centers and programs, and other community-based programs and groups. To communicate a clear message that the intervention works, the client will utilize promotional videos, host webinars for potential partners, and send animated eCards to potential partners through the client's network. Once COVID-19 gathering restrictions are lifted, the intervention will be presented at conferences, health fairs, workshops, and community events. **Dissemination channels** may include radio or TV interviews and public service announcements (PSAs), social media platforms that are most popular with youth such as Facebook, Snapchat, TikTok, and Instagram. Also, websites YouTube, print mailings, journals, reports, newsletters, and more. **What will be disseminated?** The first-ever mHealth intervention designed for youth between the ages of 15–24, builds wellness and resilience through culturally responsive messaging, role modeling, skill-building, and connections. The intervention is an evidence-based approach that addresses topics such as healthy relationships, pride, help-seeking skills, domestic violence, substance misuse, and suicidality. **How and why?** The intervention offers youth education through videos and text messaging. The intervention is easy to integrate into existing services, programs, and schools. Evaluation of the intervention with 1,044 teens and young adults nationwide show that it was effective, and improved health behaviors, resilience, positive coping, self-efficacy, and self-esteem. **Dissemination partners**: Partners can help disseminate the intervention. Current partnerships include programs, projects funded by the Substance Abuse and Mental Health Administration, the Department of Education, and many others. Utilizing the reach of partners through their social media platforms, listservs, websites, collaborators will increase the reach of intervention dissemination efforts. **Reaching partners and potential partners**: Marketing strategies include creating intervention social media awareness through promotional videos or clips, hosting webinars for potential partners, and sending materials such as animated eCards to raise awareness through avenues such as listservs. Once COVID-19 gathering restrictions are lifted, the client will promote the intervention at conferences and workshops to extend influence. Presenting at conferences and workshops, social media, emails, video text messaging, and encouraging abstract submissions for promoting the intervention at conferences will extend influence. **Reaching end-users:** Broadcast media offers several platforms to promote the intervention, such as radio or TV interviews and PSAs, social media platforms that are most popular with youth such as Facebook, Snapchat, TikTok, and Instagram, partner websites, YouTube, mailings, journals, reports, and newsletters. Personal connections that can be utilized include professional networks, workshops, existing grants and program efforts, academic partnerships and their networks, and others. **Potential barriers** include the ability to market the intervention on a broader scale, such as through conference opportunities. Also, limited buy-in from potential youth to attend the series due to lack of information or access. Internet services may be severely limited to non-existent in some areas. Barriers can be overcome by relying on established partners to raise awareness of the intervention through their social media platforms. Then the intervention can utilize youth and partner input to create buzz on various social media platforms, such as Snapchat, Instagram, and TikTok, to reach the target population. Programs can create wi-fi "hot spots" offering the series for youth, and these hot spots can provide iPads or computers for youth to view sessions. **Evaluation:** Evaluating the effectiveness of the dissemination strategy may occur in the future. This may include the number of partners reached, intervention promotional video views and reactions, number of website hits, number of inquiries that the client receives about the intervention, number of printed and electronic eCards distributed and reactions to these, and qualitative data from the client on successes and challenges about disseminating the intervention throughout the United States. Evaluation may also capture new and existing partners that contact the client for more information, and the actual number of partners who implement the intervention. **Dissemination methods:** This includes the method, frequency, and audience. Examples of dissemination methods here include newsletter, website, press releases, flyers, meetings, postcards, social media, conferences and presentations, workshops, journal articles, reports, and other documents and methods as required. **Frequency** of dissemination is daily, weekly, monthly, quarterly, annually, or as needed. **Every day** check and update postings, reply to comments and questions, monitor the intervention online mentions, monitor trending hashtags, monitor comments. **Every week** create a posting schedule for the week, track results of social media campaigns. **Every month** collect stats, research news, and topics that can be used to promote the intervention, apply the previous month's success to a future month. **Every quarter** review and evaluate the last quarter, make sure the intervention brand image is consistent across social medial channels, conduct audience analysis to ensure targets are appropriate, set goals for next quarter. **Every year** update dissemination strategy, evaluate efforts, refine, and implement. Examples of audiences include partners, staff, youth, policymakers, researchers, funding agencies, or everyone.

Social Media and Messaging

We use social media more than we did a month ago, or even a year ago. Social media has the power to transform and reach more people than traditional marketing methods. When developing a social media communication plan, consider the people that you want to reach, the objectives of the social media approach, your goals (specific and measurable is always good), a summary of content, and frequency of content. Box 7.1 is an example of a communication plan that utilizes print and social media strategies that could be adapted for any program or community.

You may also consider being more specific in your approach. We work with several programs that have Facebook pages. List the names of Facebook pages that will be managed (some have more than one and open or closed groups). **Consider who you will reach**: This might be individuals in recovery, family members, professionals, leaders, educators, artists, advocates, youth service professionals, and others on Facebook who like the organization. **Target goals** and benefits should explain who will be reached and the reason, for example, the Facebook page will reach community members who are isolated due to COVID-19 and provide unique information about recovery that can't be found anywhere else. **Target velocity** is another area to consider, how frequently will you post content. This might be every morning with the morning meditation and monitoring conversations and discussions throughout the day. **Formats** include the types of content that will be posted, some examples include videos, posters, photos with quotes of inspiration. **Tone and rules of engagement** should also be established. An example is, content must be less than 280 characters, videos play automatically, communication emphasizes visuals over text. **Resources required** to outline what is needed. This might include who is in charge of managing the page and communications, who is authorized to post content, and the contact person if people have questions or if issues arise. Key performance indicators for Facebook might include the number of views, shares, likes, discussions, and other metrics to gauge content performance against goals.

SAMSHA and other organizations developed evidence-based (tested and true) social media toolkits for treatment programs (and others) to use on social media. Check out the Resources section at the end of this chapter for more

Box 7.1   Communication Plan Template for Recovery Treatment

People We Want to Reach

- New and existing recovery clients living in _____ and beyond.
- Families seeking information about recovery and wellness.
- Community members interested in supporting recovery and participating in events.
- Leaders and policymakers leading recovery initiatives.

Objectives

- Expand access to community recovery resources and opportunities for people from all walks of life in _____ and beyond.
- Support outreach and education about recovery and wellness collaborative partnerships and training.
- Promote evidence-based best practice interventions that build on strengths and resiliency to promote wellness in _____ and beyond.

Goals

- Reach #____ individuals using Facebook, Instagram, and YouTube channels monthly. Increase number of followers on each platform by 20% annually— Facebook current #____, 20% increase #____, Instagram current #____, 20% increase #___, YouTube current # ___, and 20% increase #___.
- Website analytics show 30% increase in views annually (current #____ and 30% increase #___).
- Reach #___, 10% increase #_____ in individuals that receive email communications about activities and trainings.
- Reach #___, 20% increase #____in printed flyers disseminated.

Content

- Electronic flyers about upcoming trainings posted at offices and partner office locations.
- Electronic versions of printed flyers on trainings will be posted to the website and updated regularly.
- Email communications to community members and partners on upcoming trainings sent monthly.
- Oral presentations (with flyers/information) during recovery month and regularly throughout the year (in-person and Zoom based on COVID-19 restrictions).

Frequency of Content

- Printed flyers and PDF electronic versions posted monthly or as needed.
- Weekly updates on Facebook, Instagram, YouTube, and website.
- Email communications weekly or as needed.
- Oral presentations weekly or monthly based on speaker availability and demands.

information. Remember, there are resources available to you and to programs that do not need to be created, you can borrow, adapt, and share what has already been developed. Why not?

Once you have developed a communication plan and you know how you intend to use social media as a platform for dissemination, **evaluate your approach**. Here is a simple summary of a Facebook page reach (these are excellent process-related data that can be used in all types of evaluations). A treatment program Facebook page has 416 followers as of August 24, 2021. Thirty new followers joined the page in the last 30 days. Sixty posts were published, this was a 10% decrease in posts from previous months. Overall, posts reached 3,679 people during the previous 30 days, this was a 23% decrease. There were 563 post engagements, this was down 10% from the previous month. The most popular Facebook post in the previous month was the Recovery Month Video with 2,291 engagements.

Public Health Takeaway—Communicating evaluation results must be a priority. Create a communication and dissemination plan and consider diverse audiences, equitable access to technology and resources, and health literacy (steps 3–4).

Bad Examples

We can learn from bad examples of social media and communication campaigns that failed. **The National Youth Anti-Drug Media Campaign** was implemented from 1999 to 2004 with three cohorts of youth between the ages of 9 and 18 years old. A theme throughout this campaign was to emphasize a youth brand phrase through something like, *Basketball: My Anti-Drug*. These campaign ads were updated throughout the campaign to focus on specific drugs like marijuana. The goal was to educate youth in America about illegal drug use and prevent initiation of use. Another goal was to get occasional users to stop using. The nationally representative sample was surveyed four different times throughout the study after exposure to the Media Campaign. There were no significant effects (Hornik et al., 2008). This $1billion effort did not work, the evaluation told us so. What if this campaign and others were never evaluated? We would continue to implement programs that do not affect outcomes.

A bit closer to home here. **The Montana Meth Project** was one that I participated in, well at least as a supporter and advocate. If you have never been to Montana, the roads are open and wide. You can drive for miles, sometimes hundreds of miles without seeing a person, another car, or a town. Imagine driving down those roads and seeing that billboard or hearing the radio ads—it is something I can still remember. Students and communities that I worked with in Montana were part of this huge public awareness campaign to address high rates of methamphetamine use. The Montana Meth Project aimed to increase perceived risk and decrease perceived benefit, promote dialogue about meth between parents and teens, and stigmatize use (if you are making and using meth, this should be viewed as socially unacceptable) (Anderson, 2010). A primary element of the project was creating advertisements that depicted meth users as dirty, dangerous, and undesirable characters. Campaign ads were aired on radio, television, and printed mediums like newspapers and billboards across the state. This campaign was the biggest on record in Montana with 45,000 television ads, 35,000 radio ads, 10,000 print impressions, and 1,000 billboards (Anderson, 2010). And naturally I thought the campaign was effective. But, like all public health efforts that are worthwhile, the project was evaluated using a fairly rigorous quasi-experimental study with non-randomized cases and controls. Controls were individuals not exposed to the campaign based on existing treatment data admissions and state survey data collected prior to the study. **Findings from this evaluation show that the Montana Meth Project had no impact on meth use.** Researchers and policymakers call for future work that explores determinants of meth use in youth. I would add a public health approach to the design, implementation, and evaluation of campaigns like this one.

Public Health Takeaway—We must consider how to evaluate our communication efforts, but we cannot evaluate everything. We create and invest in products but we never really know how many people read them, how these reports make them feel, and what the value and impact of the products are. Marketing campaigns have the potential to reach millions, it is imperative that the message we send targets the knowledge, attitudes, and beliefs of the audience we intend to reach.

Beware of Quantification Bias

I am a researcher. I am an evaluator. I love data and I love numbers, perhaps you do as well. There is nothing like being able to ask a question and have a clear undisputable answer. "How many days in the past 30 did you attend a recovery support meeting?" Answer, 5 days. There, we have it. We know the person attended meetings on five of the last 30 days. But why did they attend the meetings, what happened when they showed up, and how did these meetings make them feel. Those are the questions that cannot always be quantified.

As a society, we love to quantify problems. As a writer, I love to quantify problems, just look at Chapter 1, the wicked problems, the prevalence of addiction, the significant percentage of people that never seek treatment ... the numbers. What if recovery is happening in a non-quantifiable way? What if evaluators and researchers need to step into qualitative and metaphysical realms to explore and observe recovery? I cannot measure or quantify what it is like to feel prayers from others, but I know in my spirit that they are there. I cannot explain to you the pull or connection that I feel toward recovery in a numerical way, but it is there. Remember the butterfly effect and chaos theory I mentioned in Chapter 2? These hold true for me, and hopefully for you.

Some stories, such as those published by Green and colleagues of spiritual awakening in natural recovery, are difficult to quantify (Green et al., 1998). Evidence, from spiritual awakenings, may not require evaluation, stories are evidence that stand alone and on their own.

Many Paths

The theories, models, and frameworks about addiction are all right and all wrong. I was thinking about this as I wrote Chapter 2 and Chapter 6. Millions of theories, models, ideas. New every decade, or even every year. I cannot keep up with all of them. Which one sticks? Which one will you pledge your practice to? In Chapter 6, I asked you to agree, for just a while, that all theories are right, true, and backed by evidence. This was a big ask, but if we are too busy thinking about our differences, who is right and wrong, and what is just and fair, we might miss an opportunity to transform what we think we know about addiction, treatment, and recovery.

Addiction and behavioral theories remind me of the religions of the world. You may be atheist (without god), Buddhist, Mormon, Catholic, Baptist, Hindu ... all of these religions work for the people that follow them. Every day in the pew, or every Tuesday in the confession room, or meditating and chanting, people have found their religions, and religions have found them. Now, if you have gone down the path of trying to find a perfect religion then you might already know that you decide what to take and what to leave. You might believe most of it, but there could be some things that do not and will never make sense, for example, why there is not a woman priest or gender equality.

Natural Recovery

I know this is a book about evaluating treatment programs, but I must add the concept of natural recovery. **Natural recovery** from alcohol and drug-use-related programs without treatment includes maturing out, auto remission, spontaneous remission, and spontaneous recovery. Most individuals with addiction do not seek help from treatment providers (Klingemann & Sobell, 2001). Harvard researchers report that 80% of individuals with AUD in recovery for more than one year did not seek or receive professional treatment (Harvard Medical School Publishing Group, 1995). Researchers in Canada found a high prevalence of recovery in untreated individuals with 77% in a national survey reporting recovery without receiving treatment (Sobell et al., 1996). Other research on alcoholism found that a significant number of people recovered without treatment or 12-step programs (Vallant, 2009). Empirical evidence has emerged challenging the disease model by demonstrating that, on average, over half of individuals recover from addiction (White, 2012; Sheedy & Whitter, 2009), many without clinical interventions.

I am sorry. Treatment programs and public health experts do not hold the keys to recovery. We do not get to decide who recovers and who does not. Individuals hold their own keys and create their conceptual doors about the recovery process (Humphreys, 2015). Humphreys writes about this in his reflection about the gatekeeper myth in public policy, attitudes, and our personal lives. At a policy level, the gatekeeper myth perpetuates the idea of a huge unmet need for treatment with just 10% of the population receiving the treatment they need, this means 90% of people still need treatment. Treatment programs want more funding to meet this treatment need, but this fails to acknowledge all of the other ways that people recover, beyond formal treatment. Why not fund art programs, rat parks, drum circles, recovery housing, mindfulness retreats, employment, and educational programs? A key issue with the concept of treatment and recovery is that when it occurs naturally, it is not necessarily reported or quantified as evidence. Remember the Cochrane Review and EBPs from Chapter 2? This virtually means that there is an entire pandora box of approaches to recovery that occur outside treatment programs.

Public Health Takeaway—Concepts of natural recovery should be recognized beyond the treatment program milieu, where recovery, treatment, and life happens outside of the bounded environment (remember our systems theory approach from Chapter 2).

Hope

When I think about hope, what gives me hope and a theory of hope I must share. Our team actually revisited the Theory of Change (ToC) model and decided to call it a Theory of Hope. We did this because it is easy to focus on what needs to change, what is wrong, and what will improve as a result of our efforts (prevention, treatment, recovery, etc.), https://aea365.org/blog/ipe-tig-week-intentionally-reframing-logic-to-hope-by-dyani-bingham-desiree-restad-kelley-milligan-and-allyson-kelley/. But an overreliance on the ToC can make us forget about what comes before change, and that is hope. Hope is the vehicle that gets us in the front seat of the car. Hope allows us to look out the window and see possibilities of what life could be like, without drugs, alcohol, depression, anxiety, shame, guilt, etc. Hope is the feeling that we get when we are inspired, connected, and supported. Here is hope for the recovery generation.

People that have been through it, through systems of racism, discrimination, criminalization, and trauma, they give me **hope that change is possible**, because **they are still here.**

Peers with the lived experience of recovery earning their certification as peer recovery support specialists, this gives me hope about systems change.

Parents getting their children back after years of being apart, the parent recovers from SUD, the children return home, this gives me hope for future generations.

Communities and leaders within those **communities investing** in the people, the people who have not been able to recover, yet the communities rally to support them, this gives me hope in the model of community.

The friend completing her 17th try at 90-day Level 3.0 treatment, her **persistence gives me hope**.

The family member who died from cirrhosis of the liver at 52, the letter that he wrote to my dad before he died, outlining his journey through addiction. The story that he drank alcohol his entire adult life ... there was only one period in his life he remembered being sober, it was for three weeks. He was violently sick these weeks away from alcohol, but he did this alone. His letter gives me hope that **others will not suffer** in the same way.

The husband who committed suicide after a lifetime of drinking, the family takes a stand to never allow drugs or alcohol in their home, this might **break the cycle**, it gives me hope.

The young man with SUD who naturally recovered, his family removed all of the alcohol from their house, they no longer drink for him. He bought a new truck, and his **partner supports him** in his new job and in his sobriety, this shows me that **employment gives people meaning and purpose**.

The grandmother who takes care of her grandchildren because the parents are on the streets, using, she is **tired and overwhelmed but continues**.

The mother who loses her daughter to a drug overdose in a motel room, **she finds a way to live** without her, but does not drive by the motel where it happened, it is too much, even after 20 years.

A man has five years of sobriety, his 10-year old daughter is diagnosed with a rare form of cancer, and she dies suddenly, and he **maintains recovery** even when tragedy strikes.

The woman who has advanced stage cirrhosis with just weeks to live enrolls in a college program to finally get the degree she has been working toward her entire life. She dies before she earns the degree, **she was determined**.

The **community that rallies** around a family impacted by addiction, giving them a **place to stay, food, clothes** ... hope abounds.

The mom wants to see her son's last basketball game of the season. He tells her she can go to the game if she shows up sober. She manages for the day and sits in the bleachers **cheering him on**.

A couple **adopts a baby** with severe fetal alcohol effect, this gives me hope.

The landlord who accepts an applicant with multiple felony drug convictions, he **takes a chance** on another person's recovery.

The client who walks through the doors of a treatment program for the first time in 20+ years of using heroin. The client completes an intake, attends their first meeting, and leaves feeling like recovery is possible. The following day the client overdoses on heroin laced with fentanyl. Staff at the treatment program are ready for the next person to come, the **doors are always open**. This gives me hope.

The staff running the needle exchange program in a rural New Mexico town, open 24 hours a day and 7 days a week. Enduring harsh words at the grocery store and glares because some do not agree with the harm reduction model, **this is strength**.

What gives you hope? Someone once told me that hope is really all there is. The older I get, the more that I believe this.

Spiritual Foundations

You might be wondering how we moved from Chapter 1, quantifying the problem to Chapter 7, talking about spirituality. I am not here to convert, but I must share the good news. We are spirits, and we live in a body. I believe that most significant experiences in life have a spiritual component. The spirit is the force that is moving me through this world and to write here today. Some people call the greater spirit God, Creator, Divine, Allah, and many other names.

It is Sunday. The book is due to Routledge tomorrow and there is just too much left to do. I've always thought about the spiritual foundations of recovery. Do people feel the spirit, their spirit, a connection to a higher power in the pew on Sunday morning at church? When do they feel like a spiritual being? Do they feel spirit wandering through a forest or on top of a mountain that overlooks a turquoise lake (we have them in Oregon).

I was meeting with an elder a few months ago. We started talking about life and family members who are struggling. I mentioned a relative that is deep in addiction. I asked the elder what could be done, and why this was happening. Her response was something that I will take with me. She said, some people are one-dimensional, they are just concerned with one thing, when people are living in a one-dimensional state the spiritual realm is not accessible to them.

What I know is that most people I have met that are in long-term recovery talk about a spiritual transformation that occurred, belief in an unseen and higher power. If you are familiar with 12-step programs (discussed throughout this text) then you know that these were created based on Christian values and biblical perspectives (the Oxford Group) (Galanter, 2007).

Brown and colleagues write about spirituality and recovery in their work, where spirituality may be conceptualized based on social connections, meaning and purpose, relationships, awareness, and beliefs in higher powers (2019). They developed a framework (I know another one) for exploring the role of spirituality in recovery from SUD (Brown et al., 2019). This new framework, spirituality in recovery or SIR asserts that spirituality is a means of converting person values into actionable behaviors. This makes sense to me. The second assertion is that the resulting healthy behaviors will lead to a recovery path and help individuals as they deal with personal problems and conflicts that may take them away from their recovery. They call for research that operationalizes spirituality to better understand the spiritual foundations of recovery.

We did not review every prevention, intervention, or recovery activity in this text because we simply ran out of time and room. But there are a few **activities that advocate for spiritual foundations** of recovery that I must include.

Green and colleagues explored stories from treatment center participants in the program to explore spiritual foundations of recovery (Green et al., 1998). Participants identified faith or the need to believe in something that cannot be seen, as a significant requirement for change and recovery. They report that one person said, "… . You have to believe in something. You can't have faith and not believe. You have faith to believe you can recover. You can't recover if you don't have faith that you can recover. That doesn't work. You have to have faith that you can recover" (1998, p. 328).

Dan Dickerson is an American Indian Psychologist that developed Drum-Assisted Recovery Therapy for Native Americans (DARTNA). Previous work has **demonstrated positive physical and psychological effects associated with drumming**. Many view drumming as a pathway toward healing, and a way to connect and build community. Some have told me that the drum is the heartbeat of the community or nation. Dickerson and his colleagues evaluated drumming, indeed this shows that everything can be evaluated. They developed a pretest with 10 Native patients with histories of SUD. Three focus groups documented perspectives from participants, providers, and the DARTNA advisory board. **Results** from their evaluation show the positive effects of drumming on spirit, mood, education, and community connections. Dickerson and colleagues write about one participant's experiences, "…I felt like I was equal in the spirit, of everybody. They were taking time out of their lives, I was too, so we had consensus right there, and we're sitting around the drum and that's why the spirit works when we're all together."

Art therapy, like it sounds, is creating art. As therapy, this targets individuals with trauma, illness, and those seeking recovery. In my work, I have witnessed the powerful impacts of art, give someone a box of crayons and a big sheet of white paper and ask them to draw something that represents how they are feeling. Often these drawings tell stories that words never could. In other cases, I have witnessed the therapeutic effects of beading, sewing, painting, storytelling, videography, photography, medicinal plant preparation, embroidery, and drum making. All of these are various forms of art therapy. Researchers promote art therapy in treatment settings for its ability to promote emotional expression, encourage spiritual recovery, and illicit creative expression (Holt & Kaiser, 2009). Holt and colleagues created the First Step Series as an approach to implementing art therapy based on Prochaska's stages of change model (Prochaska & DiClemente, 1983; Prochaska & Norcross, 2001). Using principles of motivational interviewing and the stages of change, Holt and colleagues asked clients to draw images of certain life events that brought them to treatment, for example, draw the crisis that brought them to treatment (this might be asked during the first session) (2009). Another art exercise is asking clients to draw a bridge of where they have been and where they want to be in relation to their recovery. A final example is to ask clients to create a cost-benefits collage that asks them to explore the costs and benefits of staying as they are or moving toward change and recovery. Sharp conducted a literature review of art therapy and recovery for individuals with physical and psychological illnesses (Sharp, 2018). Her findings suggest that art therapy is beneficial for people in recovery. It's time for art.

Mindfulness: Garland and colleagues explored mindfulness-oriented recovery enhancement for chronic pain and prescription opioid misuse in a randomized control trial (RCT) (2014). They randomized 115 patients with chronic pain into a treatment and control group (Garland et al., 2014) and assessed outcomes at pre- and post-treatment, and 3 months after the intervention. They explored changes in opioid use status and desire for opioids, stress, non-reactivity, and reappraisal. **Findings** from their RCT demonstrate the feasibility and efficacy of mindfulness as an effective approach and treatment for addressing co-occurring prescription opioid misuse, stress, and chronic pain.

Integrated approaches that incorporate aspects of spirituality can be effective. Atkins called for integrative approaches that include cognitive-behavioral therapies, peer recovery support, mindfulness, dialectical behavior therapy, trauma treatment, wellness treatments, and family works. Wellness strategies could include exercise, sleep hygiene, prayer, meditation, nutrition, and mind–body techniques. Family efforts include education, groups, family therapy, and specific interventions when appropriate (Atkins, 2018). There are more.

The Future

We are getting near the end.

What We Still Know

We started this text with a review of the current MHSUD epidemic, crisis, emergency. We reviewed frameworks, models, and approaches designed to address the current crisis. What we know now—the epidemic, increasing rates of SUD and MI are due to context and conditions. Unequal distribution of impacts due to social status. Minority populations have been hit the hardest. Evaluators often work on the ground, side-by-side, with communities and treatment programs. Evaluators witness all forms of health and healthcare disparities, inequities, and inequalities. One glaring disparity from the National Institute on Minority Health and Health Disparities is that just 10% of individuals with a mental health disorder receive effective treatment (National Institutes of Health, 2015). Disparities and inequities are often rooted in oppression, racism, and discrimination (National Academies of Sciences et al., 2019). All are barriers for individuals, families, and communities reaching their highest level of health and wellbeing. Data collected during the COVID-19 pandemic show that people of color experienced greater physical and mental health disparities during the pandemic, and Black and American Indian or Alaska Native groups ranked the worst (Henry et al., 2020). Perhaps, this is not a surprise to health advocates, researchers, evaluators, and policymakers… but it needs to change. One of the greatest injustices that evaluators often report is the limited access to mental health services for individuals in need, and the lack of recognition that mental health is just as important as our physical health. Can you imagine emergency rooms turning away someone with an open fracture, or a bone sticking out of the skin? I cannot. Yet our healthcare system makes people wait up to 6 months when they are in crisis and need immediate mental health services. A few weeks ago, I was talking with some of the communities that I work in, the treatment programs and youth-serving organizations. In one community, they said it takes 182.5 days to get a mental health appointment scheduled another community said it was 91.2 days. Public health urges us not to just sit with these glaring disparities but do something about them. One example of how communities are addressing these injustices is through legislation. For example, California's Senate Bill 221 will reduce the wait times for mental health appointments and require providers to see individuals within 10 business days (*California - SB-221 Health Care Coverage: Timely Access to Care.*, n.d.). Similarly, Montana is advocating for legislation that addresses mental health professional shortage areas by adjusting standards for licensing psychologists from other states to move to Montana (*Montana SB90 | 2021 | Regular Session*, n.d., p. 90). California and Montana are leading the way for mental health and social justice in the west.

What are the overall key public health takeaways and messages that we must carry forward? Here are some of my ideas.

Message 1—Researchers and Evaluators Unite with Evidence

Evaluation inside of treatment programs is happening all the time. Publications about the effects of interventions, what works, what does not, for whom, and why are not always published or readily available. In Chapter 2, we reviewed differences in research and evaluation, we glimpsed at the similarities, and even considered the notion that we possibly walk in both worlds. We do. Researchers in the United States and beyond belong to an elite group. With PhDs, MDs, and various graduate degrees, researchers have privilege, power, access, and expectations about their scholarship. Researchers may have specific ideas about their contributions to the literature, the kinds of scientific evidence they generate, and the articles and journals they publish in. I would argue that evaluators are often in the back seat. I can say this because I walk in both worlds, you might too. Some evaluators do not have the doctoral training, NIH researcher status, institutional support, or a small nation of graduate assistants stepping up to do the groundwork. But I believe that evaluators belong to an elite group as well. Evaluators deserve a seat at the table, an opportunity to publish their work, a competitive chance at any NIH R01 research proposal, and more. It is time that researchers and evaluators come together about publication and dissemination. We have a ton of evidence about what works and what does not. Sometimes evidence never gets into the hands of the people that need it most. We continue to do the same things, the same treatment, the same cycle, and they may not work.

Alternatively, sometimes we have evidence, like that from the Montana Meth Project, that tells us that a certain intervention or campaign is not effective. These results are published in accessible journals, and people like you and me read the results and think, wow, I had no idea.

This is the call. We cannot write a report and file it in a box and move on to the next big thing. The public and seven future generations deserve to know what we found, even if the findings do not support our goals and objectives, or the desired outcomes of a given project. When thinking about the evaluation approach, always consider the critical evaluation question, "What did you find that could help others? Improve treatment programs? Effectiveness? Community support? Build equity?"

Message 2—Substance Use is the Most Visible Addiction

Addiction is a brain disease. Addiction is also a community and family disease. Addiction is a societal disease. Addiction is not just about abusing alcohol and drugs; these are simply the most visible forms of addiction in our world. Addiction does not discriminate based on race, ethnicity, gender, sexual orientation, or geography, it is everywhere and in every community.

People are suffering. They want to heal. Funding must be readily available to aggressively treat addiction, just like any other diseases we would treat in our healthcare system or outside of the healthcare system. Behavioral health integration in healthcare cannot wait any longer, the time is now (National Academies of Sciences et al., 2019). At the same time, we must recognize the fact that the majority of individuals with MHSUD recover without clinical interventions or in a treatment setting. This means that we must expand our thinking and ideas about recovery beyond the disease-based pathology (Lewis, 2017).

Message 3—Policy Change is the Path Forward

Policy change cannot happen soon enough. I am encouraged by the proposed legislation that will fund mental health, increase access to MAT providers, and reduce wait times to access treatment services. But I cannot believe how incredibly slow all of this is. If a bill was proposed in 2019, why are we still waiting? One of the key issues moving forward with policy is the politics and economics that drive policy uptake. We have presented several key policy issues in this text, and specifically in Chapter 6. Current public policies are failing mankind. Policy change is slow, it takes time, and it is not for the faint at heart, but it is worth it. Do you enjoy flying on an airplane without the person next to you smoking a cigarette? What about age requirements that prevent your 13-year-old daughter from walking into a store and purchasing alcohol or cigarettes? How about the ability to access treatment and mental health services and have your insurance pay for it? If you see the value in these things, thank public health policy advocates and developers.

Message 4—Conditions Create Problems

What if addiction (MHSUD) is not the problem? What if we have been targeting the wrong outcomes all along? What if it is the conditions that are the problem? It's possible that we as a society have created unhealthy forests and soil that force people to cope in dangerous ways? Remember the Rat Park experiments? What about recovery housing and housing first models? What if the recovery generation is one that normalizes abstinence, promotes addiction as a treatable condition, talks openly and vulnerably about the issues, and more importantly takes action.

Message 5—Evaluation to Promote Social Justice

Some of the most glaring injustices are occurring with people of color in the United States and beyond. The current pandemic has not made these injustices disappear, they are worse. A public health approach requires a focus on equity and justice. What are you willing to do in your work and life right now that promotes justice? Equitable access to treatment? End discrimination and racism? One of my teachers told me that social justice is a spiritual act. I have been thinking about this for a while now. I agree. To be concerned about social justice, and to do something requires a level of self-awareness and compassion that not everyone has developed (yet). What stage of readiness do you find yourself in? Are readers, evaluators, researchers, policymakers just in the stage of precontemplation (Prochaska & Norcross, 2001). Maybe you read this book, you are just at the first stage of wanting to change a behavior, change your evaluation practices, change how you view harm reduction models, change how you think about the theory of change and theory of hope. This is your invitation, now is your time.

Public Health Takeaway—Addiction is everywhere. It is not just about drugs and alcohol; it is about not being present in a world full of possibilities and hope. Addiction takes us away from those possibilities and impacts everyone. Recovery brings us back into the sacred circle of life.

Heal

We carry our ancestors with us, their DNA, their stories and histories, the good and the bad. Two days before the submission deadline for this book I decided to treat myself to a one-hour acupuncture visit. I started acupuncture treatment several years ago when I had severe migraines and tendonitis, this was the only thing that relieved my pain. After those two issues resolved, I continued acupuncture treatments. I do so as a preventative measure and to provide clarity in my work and my life. Sometimes during the hour-long treatment, I have visions. I see and feel things that are spiritual or metaphysical in nature. This week, I vividly saw my friends and relatives who are not here in the physical world anymore. They were sitting around a big fire; everything was dark except for the flames and their young faces. Their facial expressions told me they finally understood. Flipping through each page of this book, and absorbing its contents, smiling, and nodding their heads yes. None of them were evaluators or researchers. Most of them died too early, alcohol, drugs, unresolved trauma and poor mental health consumed them. Our world did not understand their disease, their behaviors, and choices. As I think about this vision (and I hope I have not lost you), I started to understand that maybe this book was not written for the world, students, classrooms, researchers, evaluators, treatment programs, families, and public health advocates. Maybe this book was for me. This book was my way of understanding all of the losses, the behaviors, the causes of addiction, the injustices and inequities in our world. These theories, explanations, and examples become the medicine or treatment that we need to heal.

> One proceeds in life, gains ground, reverses injustice and stands against the winds, through the strength of the spirit.
>
> Clarissa Pinkola Estes, 1996, p. 516.

Discussion Questions

1. How has this chapter and this book changed how you feel about recovery?
2. What are some challenges and potential solutions to communicating evaluation findings in your work?
3. Describe alternative approaches to healing and recovery? What are some challenges and strengths of evaluations that capture non-quantifiable meanings?
4. Think about your place in the recovery generation. Where are you? What are you compelled to do as a researcher, evaluator, student, policymaker, leader, parent? Write these actionable behaviors on a note. Look at them every day and make the choice to create a world that is better than it was yesterday.

Resources

Athena Opioid Prevention Social Media Campaign, https://theathenaforum. org/opioid-prevention-campaign-social-media-toolkit
National Institutes of Health, Heal Initiative, https://heal.nih.gov/
Starts with One Opioid Misuse Campaign, https://getthefactsrx.com/
Stephanie Evergreen, Intentional Reporting and Data Visualization, https:// stephanieevergreen.com/
Substance Abuse and Mental Health Services Administration, Opioid Overdose Prevention Toolkit, https://store.samhsa.gov/product/Opioid-Overdose-Prevention-Toolkit/SMA18-4742

References

Anderson, D. M. (2010). Does information matter? The effect of the Meth Project on meth use among youths. *Journal of Health Economics*, 29(5), 732–742. 10.1016/j.jhealeco.2010.06.005

Atkins, C. (2018). *Opioid Use Disorders: A Holistic Guide to Assessment, Treatment, and Recovery*. PESI. http://ebookcentral.proquest.com/lib/uncg/detail.action?docID=6253999

Brown, A. M., McDaniel, J. M., Austin, K. L., & Ashford, R. D. (2019). Developing the spirituality in recovery framework: The function of spirituality in 12-step substance use disorder recovery. *Journal of Humanistic Psychology*, 0022167819871742. 10.1177/0022167819871742

California SB-221 (n.d.). *Health Care Coverage: Timely Access to Care*. Retrieved November 14, 2021, from https://leginfo.legislature.ca.gov/faces/billNavClient.xhtml?bill_id=202120220SB221

Estes, C. P. (2008). *Women who run with the wolves: Contacting the power of the wild woman*. Random House.

Galanter, M. (2007). Spirituality and recovery in 12-step programs: An empirical model. *Journal of Substance Abuse Treatment*, 33(3), 265–272. 10.1016/j.jsat.2007.04.016

Garland, E. L., Manusov, E. G., Froeliger, B., Kelly, A., Williams, J. M., & Howard, M. O. (2014). Mindfulness-oriented recovery enhancement for chronic pain and prescription opioid misuse: Results from an early stage randomized controlled trial. *Journal of Consulting and Clinical Psychology*, 82(3), 448–459. 10.1037/a0035798

Green, L. L., Fullilove, M. T., & Fullilove, R. E. (1998). Stories of spiritual awakening. *Journal of Substance Abuse Treatment*, 15(4), 325–331. 10.1016/S0740-5472(97)00211-0

Harvard Medical School Publishing Group. (1995). *Treatment of Drug Abuse and Addiction - Part III*. Harvard Mental Health Letter.

Henry, B. F., Mandavia, A. D., Paschen-Wolff, M. M., Hunt, T., Humensky, J. L., Wu, E., Pincus, H. A., Nunes, E. V., Levin, F. R., & El-Bassel, N. (2020). COVID-19, mental health, and opioid use disorder: Old and new public health crises intertwine. *Psychological Trauma: Theory Research, Practice and Policy*, 12(Suppl 1), S111–S112. 10.1037/tra0000660

Holt, E., & Kaiser, D. H. (2009). The first step series: Art therapy for early substance abuse treatment. *The Arts in Psychotherapy*, 36(4), 245–250. 10.1016/j.aip.2009.05.004

Hornik, R., Jacobsohn, L., Orwin, R., Piesse, A., & Kalton, G. (2008). Effects of the national youth anti-drug media campaign on youths. *American Journal of Public Health*, 98(12), 2229–2236. 10.2105/AJPH.2007.125849

Humphreys, K. (2015). Addiction treatment professionals are not the gatekeepers of recovery. *Substance Use & Misuse*, 50(8–9), 1024–1027. 10.3109/10826084.2015.1007678

Kelley, A. (2018). *Evaluation in Rural Communities*. Routledge. 10.4324/9780429458224

Kelley, A. (2020). *Public Health Evaluation and the Social Determinants of Health* (Vol. 1–1 online resource [xi, 178 pages]: illustrations, maps). Routledge, Taylor & Francis Group. https://www.taylorfrancis.com/books/9781003047810

Klingemann, H. K., & Sobell, L. C. (2001). Introduction: Natural recovery research across substance use. *Substance Use & Misuse*, 36(11), 1409–1416. https://doi.org/10.1081/ja-100106957

Lewis, M. (2017). Addiction and the brain: Development, not disease. *Neuroethics*, 10(1), 7–18. 10.1007/s12152-016-9293-4

Montana SB90 (n.d.) *2021 Regular Session*. LegiScan. Retrieved November 14, 2021, from https://legiscan.com/MT/text/SB90/id/2247400

National Academies of Sciences, Engineering, and Medicine, Health and Medicine Division, Board on Population Health and Public Health Practice, Roundtable on Health Literacy, Wojtowicz, A., & Alper, J. (2019). *The Intersection of Behavioral Health, Mental Health, and Health Literacy: Proceedings of a Workshop*. National Academies Press. http://ebookcentral.proquest.com/lib/uncg/detail.action?docID=5746565

National Institutes of Health (2015). *10 Percent of US Adults Have Drug Use Disorder at Some Point in Their Lives*. National Institutes of Health (NIH). https://www.nih.gov/news-events/news-releases/10-percent-us-adults-have-drug-use-disorder-some-point-their-lives

Prochaska, J. O., & DiClemente, C. C. (1983). Stages and processes of self-change of smoking: Toward an integrative model of change. *Journal of Consulting and Clinical Psychology, 51*(3), 390–395. 10.1037/0022-006X.51.3.390

Prochaska, J. O., & Norcross, J. C. (2001). Stages of change. *Psychotherapy: Theory, Research, Practice, Training, 38*(4), 443–448. 10.1037/0033-3204.38.4.443

Rushing, S. C., Kelley, A., Bull, S., Stephens, D., Wrobel, J., Silvasstar, J., Peterson, R., Begay, C., Dog, T. G., McCray, C., Brown, D. L., Thomas, M., Caughlan, C., Singer, M., Smith, P., & Sumbundu, K. (2021). Efficacy of an mHealth intervention (BRAVE) to promote mental wellness for American Indian and Alaska native teenagers and young adults: Randomized controlled trial. *JMIR Mental Health, 8*(9), e26158. 10.2196/26158

Sharp, M. (2018). Art therapy and the recovery process: A literature review. *Expressive Therapies Capstone Theses*. https://digitalcommons.lesley.edu/expressive_theses/30

Sheedy, C. K., & Whitter, M. (2009). *Guiding Principles and Elements of Recovery-Oriented Systems of Care: What Do We Know From the Research?* HHS Publication No. (SMA) 09-4439. Rockville, MD: Center for Substance Abuse Treatment, Substance Abuse and Mental Health Services Administration.

Sobell, L. C., Cunningham, J. A., & Sobell, M. B. (1996). Recovery from alcohol problems with and without treatment: Prevalence in two population surveys. *American Journal of Public Health, 86*(7), 966–972. https://www.ncbi.nlm.nih.gov/pmc/articles/PMC1380437/

Vallant, G. (2009). *The Natural History of Alcoholism Revisited*. Harvard University Press. ISBN:978-0674603783

White, W. (2012). Recovery/Remission from Substance Use Disorders: An analysis of reported outcomes in 415 scientific reports, 1868-2011. Philadelphia Department of Behavioral Health and Intellectual Disability Services. http://www.williamwhitepapers.com/pr/2012%20Recovery-Remission%20from%20Substance%20Use%20DisordersFinal.pdf

Appendix A

Assessment of Recovery Capital (ARC) Instrument (Bowen et al., 2020)

The ARC can be self-administered to assess recovery using a simple scoring methodology with each subscale including five associated items at a value of **one point per item**. Each ARC subscale therefore receives a score between 0 and 5, with 5 being the highest recovery capital score within each subscale. Thus, the total ARC score is calculated out of a possible 50. This takes about 5 to 10 minutes to complete.

1. **Substance use and sobriety**

   1.1 I am currently completely sober.
   1.2 I feel I am in control of my substance use.
   1.3 I have had no "near things" about relapsing.
   1.4 I have had no recent periods of substance intoxication.
   1.5 There are more important things to me in life than using substances.
   Total Score_____

2. **Global health—psychological**

   2.1 I am able to concentrate when I need to.
   2.2 I am coping with the stresses in my life.
   2.3 I am happy with my appearance.
   2.4 In general, I am happy with my life.
   2.5 What happens to me in the future mostly depends on me.
   Total Score_____

3. **Global health—physical**

   3.1 I cope well with everyday tasks.
   3.2 I feel physically well enough to work.
   3.3 I have enough energy to complete the tasks I set myself.
   3.4 I have no problems getting around.
   3.5 I sleep well most nights.
   Total Score_____

4. Citizenship and community involvement

4.1 I am proud of the community I live in and feel part of it—sense of belonging.

4.2 It is important for me to contribute to society and or be involved in activities that contribute to my community.

4.3 It is important for me to do what I can to help other people.

4.4 It is important for me that I make a contribution to society.

4.5 My personal identity does not revolve around drug use or drinking.

Total Score_____

5. Social support

5.1 I am happy with my personal life.

5.2 I am satisfied with my involvement with my family.

5.3 I get lots of support from friends.

5.4 I get the emotional help and support I need from my family.

5.5 I have a special person with whom I can share my joys and sorrows.

Total Score_____

6. Meaningful activities

6.1 I am actively involved in leisure and sport activities.

6.2 I am actively engaged in efforts to improve myself (training, education, and/or self-awareness).

6.3 I engage in activities that I find enjoyable and fulfilling.

6.4 I have access to opportunities for career development (job opportunities, volunteering, or apprenticeships).

6.5 I regard my life as challenging and fulfilling without the need for using drugs or alcohol.

Total Score_____

7. Housing safety

7.1 I am proud of my home.

7.2 I am free of threat or harm when I am at home.

7.3 I feel safe and protected where I live.

7.4 I feel that I am free to shape my own destiny.

7.5 My living space has helped to drive my recovery journey.

Total Score_____

8. Risk-taking

8.1 I am free from worries about money.

8.2 I have the personal resources I need to make decisions about my future.

8.3 I have the privacy I need.

8.4 I make sure I do nothing that hurts or damages other people.

8.5 I take full responsibility for my actions.

Total Score_____

9. Coping and functioning

9.1 I am happy dealing with a range of professional people.
9.2 I do not let other people down.
9.3 I eat regularly and have a balanced diet.
9.4 I look after my health and wellbeing.
9.5 I meet all of my obligations promptly.
Total Score_____

10. Recovery experience

10.1 Having a sense of purpose in life is important to my recovery journey.
10.2 I am making good progress on my recovery journey.
10.3 I engage in activities and events that support my recovery.
10.4 I have a network of people I can rely on to support my recovery.
10.5 When I think of the future, I feel optimistic.
Total Score_____

Reference

Bowen, E. A., Scott, C. F., Irish, A., & Nochajski, T. H. (2020). Psychometric properties of the assessment of recovery capital (ARC) instrument in a diverse low-income sample. *Substance Use and Misuse, 55*(1), 108–118. https://doi-org.libproxy.uncg.edu/10.1080/10826084.2019.1657148

Appendix B

Confidentiality and Data Use Agreement Example

Confidentiality Agreement

I hereby acknowledge, by my signature below, that I understand that any patient information which I see or hear is considered private and confidential. I understand that confidentiality must be maintained whether the information is stored on paper or on computer, or communicated orally or through any other means.

I understand that I am not authorized to seek or deliberately obtain access to patient information. I also understand that employee information of a private or sensitive nature must also be treated as confidential, including employment records, job evaluations, etc. I have been informed that it would be illegal for me to access computerized patient or employee information without the authorization of my supervisor.

I understand that unauthorized disclosure of patient information, or any other confidential or proprietary information from this office, is unethical and/or illegal and that it is grounds for disciplinary action, up to and including my immediate dismissal from employment or termination of my contracted arrangement. All data belong to _____

I understand that this duty of confidentiality and non-disclosure will continue to apply even after I am no longer working for this office.

Name (Print)_____

Signature _____ Date: _____

Witness Signature_____ Date: _____

Title

Data Use Agreement for Accucare Access between EVALUATOR NAME or ORGANIZATION and TREATMENT PROGRAM NAME.

Parties and Purpose

This Agreement is between EVALUATOR NAME or ORGANIZATION and TREATMENT PROGRAM NAME. EVALUATOR NAME or ORGANIZATION and TREATMENT PROGRAM NAME are entering into an Agreement because that will allow the exchange of data and clarification of data access and use. TREATMENT PROGRAM NAME will provide data collected to EVALUATOR NAME or ORGANIZATION for the purposes of evaluation of TREATMENT PROGRAM NAME grant-funded initiatives.

Authority

TREATMENT PROGRAM NAME is a recovery organization whose mission is to help every person in their recovery. The authority for TREATMENT PROGRAM NAME to enter into this Agreement is NAME OF PERSON WITH AUTHORITY. This authority permits the release of data to EVALUATOR NAME or ORGANIZATION. The TREATMENT PROGRAM NAME permits disclosure of electronic health record data for evaluation functions. EVALUATOR NAME or ORGANIZATION is a small woman-owned, S Corporation whose mission is to transform communities through training, evaluation, and research at the local level.

Terms and Conditions

Description of planned data use by EVALUATOR NAME or ORGANIZATION, consistent with the Purpose above.

- Treatment of data anomalies, including technical assistance from TREATMENT PROGRAM NAME and redelivery as needed
- Terms for data storage, treatment of original data, handling of Personally Identifiable Information, and data linkage protocols
- Conditions for storing modified data (including integrated, recoded, de-identified, and derived data) during and after the project
- Terms for storage of researcher generated files (including retention/archiving, e.g., to the extent permitted by law; the original data received from TREATMENT PROGRAM NAME will be retained by EVALUATOR NAME or ORGANIZATION for ongoing periods based on evaluation contracts that require access to the electronic health record for treatment outcomes related to data.

Data Elements

The following data will be provided under this Agreement:
  Access to electronic health record database

Approved Research Uses

Document prevalence, explore risk and protective factors, document predictors of recovery outcomes, report results to TREATMENT PROGRAM NAME

Roles & Responsibilities

- TREATMENT PROGRAM NAME agrees to provide access to EVALU-ATOR NAME or ORGANIZATION to Accucare.
- TREATMENT PROGRAM NAME will comply with all applicable federal and state laws and regulations relating to the use and disclosure, the safeguarding, confidentiality, and maintenance of the data. To allow EVALUATOR NAME or ORGANIZATION to link with electronic health record data to complete their analysis.
- EVALUATOR NAME or ORGANIZATION agrees to access, hold, use, and disclose data only for the authorized uses related to evaluation. To comply with all applicable federal and state laws and regulations relating to the use and disclosure, the safeguarding, confidentiality, and maintenance of the data. To ensure that all data users comply with the requirements of this Agreement. To immediately report within 5 days any use or disclosure of Protected Data other than as expressly allowed by this Agreement. Notice shall be given to the contact _____. Any changes in the planned use of the data must be submitted to TREATMENT PROGRAM NAME in writing and receive written approval.

Duration, Amendments, and Modifications

This Agreement is effective on the date it is signed by both parties. The Agreement shall terminate annually following the date on which it becomes effective. If, at the end of the agreement, the parties wish to continue the relationship, they must execute a new Agreement.

The parties shall review this Agreement at least once every 12 months or whenever a Tribal statute is enacted that materially affects the substance of the Agreement, in order to determine whether it should be revised, renewed, or canceled.

Notwithstanding all other provisions of this Agreement, the Parties agree that

a. This Agreement may be amended at any time by written mutual consent of both parties and
b. Either party may terminate this Agreement upon thirty (30) days written notice to the other party.

Termination

Either party may terminate this Agreement for any reason on 15 business days' notice to the other party. Each party may terminate this Agreement with immediate effect by delivering notice of the termination to the other party, if the other party fails to perform, has made or makes any inaccuracy in, or otherwise materially breaches, any of its obligations, covenants, or representations, and the failure, inaccuracy, or breach continues for a period of 15 business days after the injured party delivers notice to the breaching party reasonably detailing the breach.

Ownership of Developed Intellectual Property

If either party develops any new Intellectual Property in connection with this Agreement, the parties shall enter into a separate definitive Agreement regarding the ownership of that new Intellectual Property.

Resolution of Disagreements

Should a disagreement arise on the interpretation of the provisions of this Agreement, or its amendments and/or revisions, that cannot be resolved at the operating level, the area(s) of disagreement shall be stated in writing by each party and presented to the other party for consideration. If agreement on interpretation is not reached within thirty (30) days, the parties shall forward the written presentation of the disagreement to respective higher officials for appropriate resolution.

Confidentiality and Non-disclosure

EVALUATOR NAME or ORGANIZATION shall use appropriate safeguards to protect the data from misuse and unauthorized access or disclosure, including maintaining adequate physical controls and password protections for any server or system on which these data are stored, ensuring that data are not stored on any mobile device (e.g., a laptop or smartphone) or transmitted electronically unless encrypted, and taking any other measures reasonably necessary to prevent any use or disclosure of the data other than as allowed under this Agreement. EVALUATOR NAME or ORGANIZATION shall ensure that any agents, including subcontractors, to whom it provides the data agree to the same restrictions and conditions listed in this Agreement. EVALUATOR NAME or ORGANIZATION will not attempt to identify any person whose information is contained in any data or attempt to contact those persons.

IT Security

EVALUATOR NAME or ORGANIZATION will comply with all laws applicable to the privacy or security of data received pursuant to this Agreement.

Publication/Disclosure Rules

EVALUATOR NAME or ORGANIZATION agrees not to publish any data resulting from the analysis process without express permission from TREAT-MENT PROGRAM NAME and named authorities. All data belong to TREATMENT PROGRAM NAME.

Limitations on Liability

In no event shall either party be liable to the other party under this Agreement or to any third party for special, consequential, incidental, punitive, or indirect damages, irrespective of whether such claims for damages are founded in contract, tort, warranty, operation of law, or otherwise or whether claims for such liability arise out of the performance or non-performance by such party hereunder.

Monitoring and Breach Notification

In the event of an actual or suspected security breach involving its information system(s), EVALUATOR NAME or ORGANIZATION will immediately notify TREATMENT PROGRAM NAME of the breach or suspected breach and will comply with all applicable breach notification laws. The parties agree to cooperate in any breach investigation and remedy of any such breach, including, without limitation, complying with any law concerning unauthorized access or disclosure.

Remedies in Event of Breach

The parties recognize that irreparable harm may result in the event of a breach of this Agreement. In the event of such a breach, the non-breaching party may be entitled to enjoin and restrain the other from any continued violation. This section shall survive termination of the Agreement. In the event that a breach is identified and it is determined by the non-breaching party that (a) individual or public notification is required and (b) that the requirement for notification is substantially caused by the other party, the party responsible for the breach shall be liable for the reasonable costs incurred by the other party to meet all federal and state legal and regulatory disclosure and notification requirements, including, but not limited to, costs for investigation, attorneys' fees, risk analysis, and any required individual or public notification, fines, and mitigation activities.

Signatures

_____

Name, Title TREATMENT PROGRAM NAME Date

_____

Name, Title, EVALUATOR NAME or ORGANIZATION Date

Appendix C

Scope of Work Example for ROSC
Start and End Dates
Title of Project and Organization

Name of Agency: Project Lead:
Website: Contact:

Action Steps	Timeline	Primary Responsibility	Evaluation Indicator (how you know you achieved this)
1. Hire a training coordinator for the 6-month project.			Training coordinator hired
2. Conduct a scan and asset map of existing PRS resources and identify potential participants for the 2-day workshop obtained through collaborative partnerships and consumers contacts.			Scan and asset map completed available in print and electronic formats. Comprehensive list of potential participants with contact information. VISTA volunteers will build upon the organization's resource list; finalize and print the resource list.
3. Advisory Board Meetings: Recruit peers, peer mentors, and recovery experts to the advisory board. Identify potential advisory board members through existing project stakeholders and community contacts.			Advisory Board Members Recruited and Roster Developed • Peers minimum • Peer Mentors • Recovery Experts • Native American Coalition • Community Innovations • Tribal Chemical Dependency Directors
4. Advisory Board Meetings: Bi-monthly Advisory Board Meetings			Total of 3 Advisory Board Meetings/ Total of 12 Conference Calls

(*Continued*)

Action Steps	Timeline	Primary Responsibility	Evaluation Indicator (how you know you achieved this)
scheduled; Bi-Weekly Conference Calls, emails			Completed. Documentation in the way of meeting minutes, agendas, follow-up correspondence, and written solutions to the identified project goals and objectives.
5. Advisory Board to assist with planning the 2-day workshop with stake-holders and collaborators.			Workshop Agenda includes stakeholder, collaborator, peer perspectives. Workshop Date/Venue/ DeterminedTechnology.
6. Advisory Board to assist with review of organiza-tion Peer Recovery Manual and BRSS TACS work plan.			Peer Recovery Support Manual, BRSS TACS Work plan updates.
7. Strategic communica-tions to potential work-shop participants including power point presentation, post cards, phone, email, Facebook, digital stories, and in-person meetings.			Communications Plan with Target Audience and a daily log of communications.
8. Host the 2-day Workshop/Manual available (hard copy/ electronic), CARF and/or Medicaid standards for Peer Specialists will be incorporated into agenda and manual.			Final Agenda Sign In Sheets
9. Evaluating the workshop and participant experi-ences/impact/likelihood of using PRS.			Evaluation Report available in print and electronic format.
10. Collaborations with human service tribal leaders/tribal chemical dependency depart-ments/behavioral health/economic devel-opment departments/or-ganizations/family/ others resulting in			Documentation of new collaborations with the organization and human service departments/ organizations/others. Summary of newly implemented approaches/ models of PRS that result from workshop. Follow-up

(*Continued*)

Action Steps	Timeline	Primary Responsibility	Evaluation Indicator (how you know you achieved this)
implemented peer-driven culturally based model appropriate for the target population.			communications and infrastructure development led by the organization. Increased participation and awareness in September's Recovery Month.

Appendix D

Worksheet for Social Media Communications Strategy (CDC, n.d.)

Use this worksheet to help you strategize about your audience, and the potential social media tools and channels you may want to use for your campaign or communication activity.

1. Determine your target audience on social media

   a. Describe the person(s) you want to reach with your communication; be as specific as possible.
   b. More than one audience may be listed. Include a primary and secondary (influencers) audience if appropriate. (Examples: mothers of children younger than two years living in Atlanta, pediatricians practicing in Nevada.)

2. Determine your objective(s)

   a. What do you want to achieve through your social media outreach and communication? This could include something you want your target audience to do as a direct result of experiencing the communication.
   b. Objectives may include (but are not limited to) the following: provide information, highlight a campaign, encourage a health behavior, reinforce health messages, encourage interaction, obtain feedback/ exchange ideas, collaborate with partners.
   c. Restate your objectives in SMART terms: Specific: Explain, in concrete, detailed, and well-defined terms, what exactly you are going to do for whom? Measurable: Your objectives should be quantifiable, with the source of measurement identified.

3. Define audience communication needs
   People access information in various ways, at different times of the day, and for different reasons. If possible, define your audience's needs by using market research and other data. You can use the following resources:

a. Pew Internet and American Life Project: http://www.pewinternet.org/
b. CDC eHealth Data Briefs: http://www.cdc.gov/socialmedia/Data/Briefs/index.html
c. Describe your audiences and their health information needs.

4. Integrate your communication goals with your overall objectives

   a. Describe how your social media objectives support your organization's mission and overall communication plan.
   b. How does it support other online or offline components? What events, either national, state, or local, present communication opportunities?

5. Develop key messages
   Develop the key messages based on the target audience and objectives identified.
6. Determine resources and capacity
   Determine who in your organization will be responsible for implementation and the number of hours they can allocate for content creation and maintenance.
7. Identify social media tools
   Determine what tools will effectively reach your target audience. Match the needs of the target audience with the tools that best support your objectives and resources.
8. Define Activities
   Based on all of the elements above, list the specific activities you will undertake to reach your communication goals and objectives.
9. Identify your key partners and their roles and responsibilities
10. Define Success for Evaluation
    What are your measures of success? Your measures of success may be different depending on your goals and objectives.
11. Evaluate
    Create an evaluation plan, see Chapters 5–7 for more information.

Reference

Centers for Disease Control (n.d.) *Social Medial Tools*. Retrieved November 14, 2021, from https://www.cdc.gov/socialmedia/tools/guidelines/guideforwriting.html

Appendix E

Navigating the Institutional Review Board (IRB) Process

Here is a summary of the types of questions that need to be answered when developing an application to an IRB. There are differences between research and evaluation, depending on the location and program, the evaluation may be exempted from IRB review.

Research Purpose and Need

- What is the research *type*? (quality assurance, survey, service delivery, clinical trial)
- What is the research *question*? What are the goals and objectives of the research?
- What do they want to prove or disprove (*hypothesis*)?
- What is the *need* for this research as identified in the protocol?

Data and Data Collection

- What specific kind of information or data are they seeking?
- Will the data collected be anonymous?
- How will the information be obtained? (e.g., interviews, surveys, access to previously collected data through a research project, access to individual records such as medical charts, blood or tissue samples, periodic tests conducted throughout project period)
- How will the data be maintained? (i.e., data security and confidentiality procedures)

Study Participants

- Who are the participants of this study? (e.g., adults, children under 18, elders, pregnant women, fetus, people in tribal jail, people with mental impairment, people with a certain health condition)

- How will they be identified? (e.g., tribal enrollment lists, clinic patient lists, student lists, people who belong to a defined group, people who attend a specific event)

Recruitment and Informed Consent

- How will they be recruited and by whom? (e.g., phone call, letter, by the primary care doctor during a clinic visit)
- Will informed consent be obtained?
- What does the consent process entail?
- What is the participant's compensation?

Data Analysis

- How will the data be analyzed?
- How will individual data be presented? (e.g., individual identifying information, individual non-identifying, aggregate information)
- How will tribal data be presented? (e.g., tribal identifying information, tribal non-identifying, multisite aggregate information)

Research Results

- How will the information gained be used? (e.g., publication, presentation at a conference, develop or enhance tribal health programs)
- What will be made of the data after the study?

The response to these questions will vary based on the type of study or evaluation being conducted and the level of review required. Some evaluations or studies are exempted from the IRB review process. For more information about IRBs and exemptions, review the Health and Human Services guidelines here: https://www. hhs.gov/ohrp/regulations-and-policy/decision-charts-2018/index.html

Appendix F

Guidelines for Developing an Evaluation Report

This is a summary of what to include in an evaluation report. The front or cover page should include the title and year. Subsequent pages may include contact information and the suggested citation format.

Summary

The summary is to be written at last. The summary is a concise overview of the evaluation report. The summary answers the following questions:

- What was evaluated?
- Why was the evaluation conducted?
- Who is the target population?
- What are the major findings and recommendations?
- Are there restrictions or limitations to the evaluation that should be noted?

The summary should be easy to read and avoid technical or unfamiliar terms. Insert funding, acknowledgments, staff contributions, and other introductory supplemental information here.

Table of Contents

In MS word, insert a Table of Contents by clicking on references, Table of Contents, Automatic. Insert a list of tables, figures, boxes or graphs by clicking on the Insert Table of Figures in MS Word, select Caption Label, and select Okay.

Background

The background describes the evaluation purpose and what it was designed to achieve. Provide a summary of the program. Add details based on the audience that will be reading the report. Notice the subheadings for non-technical and technical audiences. Consider the following text in the background section:

- Origin and aims of the program
- Participants in the program
- Characteristics of the program and delivery of materials, interventions, outreach, or other
- Staff involved in the program
- Organization's role in supporting the program or evaluation

Description of Evaluation

Non-technical Audience

Why was the evaluation conducted?

The evaluation description includes why the evaluation was conducted. It also includes what it was intended to accomplish. For example, was the purpose to add value, to document the process, to document the impact, or to conduct a cost-benefit analysis.

Technical Audience

For technical audiences, the description should include the following:

- Purpose of evaluation
- Evaluation design
- Outcome measures with the instrument used and data collection procedures
- Implementation measures

Results

The results section is a summary of the evaluation findings based on the purpose and outcomes. This includes text, graphs, charts, tables, and figures. This should be used to support the information presented but not as stand-alone objects. When presenting the results, consider the format of telling the reader what you want them to know, show the reader in the form of illustrations (a table or figure), tell the reader again what you want them to know.

Non-Technical Audience

Use familiar terms to describe results, define new concepts and terms when necessary. At a minimum, include how many people participated, what was the value of the program or impact, and how do the results compare to the expected outcomes? What led to these changes? How do we know these changes are the result of the program?

Technical Audience

Cover the following in the results section for technical audiences:

- Results of the evaluation
- How many people or organizations participated?
- What were the short-, medium-, and long-term impacts from the program on participants or organizations?
- How do participants compare to other groups if data are available?
- Did participants, organizations, or other areas change as a result of the program? If yes, what led to these changes.
- Are the differences in results statistically significant?

Limitations

Present limitations of the evaluation and consider readability for non-technical audiences. Non-technical audiences may prefer the term weaknesses rather than limitations. In some instances, the limitations section may not be appropriate for non-technical audiences. Common limitations in the evaluation include small numbers or sample size, difficulty comparing results to other populations and contexts, convenience sampling methods, use of self-report data, misclassification and underreporting of minority status, linking program activities to outcomes, and others.

Discussion

Non-Technical Audience

What do the results mean?

Technical Audience

Interpret the evaluation findings based on evaluation goals and the purpose of the evaluation. At a minimum the discussion should include the following:

- Other possible explanations for results documented
- If results are generalizable
- Strengths and weaknesses of the program
- Unexpected results

Cost and Benefits

The cost-benefit section is optional and should only be included if it was part of the evaluation plan. There are several different types of cost-benefit analysis evaluation and the information to include will vary. Generally, cost-benefit analysis evaluations include the following:

- The method used to calculate the costs and benefits
- How costs and outcomes were defined in the evaluation plan?
- Costs of the program
- Benefits associated with the program
- Measures of effectiveness
- Unexpected benefits

Conclusion

Non-technical and Technical Audience

The conclusion section includes clear and concise recommendations. Write the most important information at the beginning of the conclusion. Include the following text in the conclusion:

Major conclusions of the evaluation
Recommendations based on results
Implications for future work, policy, funding, education, and others

Appendixes

Provide data tables and other supporting information from the report based on the evaluation results. Include evaluation instruments used, data collection procedures, storage, and approvals.

Technical Audience Only

- Assessments on the validity and reliability of measures
- Explanations of units of measurement
- Treatment of nonresponse items and missing values, and if imputations were made
- Response rates, assessment of nonresponsive bias, and weighting if used
- Descriptive statistics
- Bivariate correlations
- Detailed statistical results and models
- Assessment of assumptions, for example, outliers and if distributions are normal
- Data transformations (to remove outliers, create indexes and scales, and results of statistics that were transformed to test assumptions)
- Strengths and weaknesses of the research design, data, and methods

Note

Add supplemental information or sources for other materials cited as footnotes.

Reference

List of all works consulted AMA 10th Edition Style or other style guides as appropriate.

Index

Pages in *italics* refer to figures, bold refer to tables, and those followed by b refer to boxes

Printed in the United States
by Baker & Taylor Publisher Services

Printed in the United States
by Baker & Taylor Publisher Services